The C.Y. O'Connor ERADE Village Foundation

Incorporating the Immunogenetics Research Foundation and the Institute of Molecular Genetics and Immunology Incorporated

E*ducation*, **R***esearch* **and D***evelopment*, **E***mployment*

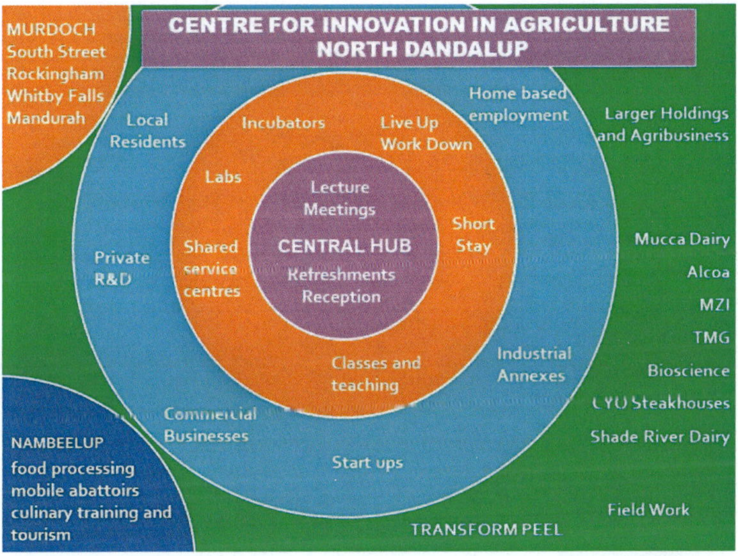

35th Annual Report 2018

C Y O'Connor ERADE Village Foundation Inc.

Employment Research and Development
Employment Technology Incubator

Street Address	24 Genomics Rise Piara Waters WA 6112
Postal Address	PO Box 5100 Canning Vale South WA 6155
Telephone	(+61 8) 9397 1556

Key Contact	Professor Roger Dawkins
Position	Chairman
Email	rldawkins@cyo.edu.au
Second Contact	Dr Sally Lloyd
Email	slloyd@cyo.edu.au

Company Overview: CYO 'Connor ERADE Village Foundation seeks to harness the intellect of young Australian post graduates whilst maintain extensive collaboration with leading institutes overseas.

Recently expanding into multidisciplinary science in fields such as bioenergy, information technology, natural products, recycling and water, the core technology is interrogation of genetic information.

The aims include understanding of human evolution in the context of disease including retroviruses, identification of new genetic markers via genomic prospecting and development of diagnostic tests for inherited traits in numerous species of medical and commercial interest such as cattle, dogs, fish and invertebrates.

Product/Service Information: The CY O'Connor Education Research and Development Employment (ERADE Village) Foundation is a charitable Foundation that conducts independent and sponsored research.

Fellowships are awarded to outstanding researchers to assist them in commercialisation of their R&D.

Published by Nearurban LLC, 1603 LBJ Freeway,
Suite 280, Dallas, TX 75234
Tel (972) 974 7130, Fax (214) 393-4001
Email : admin@nearurban.net

Manufactured and printed by CreateSpace.

ISBN: 978-0-9864115-5-7

Title and Cover image:

NU Publishing

FRIENDS OF CYO'CONNOR VILLAGE

The Foundation is a charitable organisation supporting education, research and development and employment. Without the help of friends of the Foundation it would not be possible to achieve all these objectives, including exciting new scientific discoveries. The Board thanks its many friends for their generous donations, bequests, collaborations, advice and assistance.

I/we (Name/s) .... (Tel)...............

Of (Address).. wish to:

Join the "Friends of CYO" ($55.00 pa) $................

Receive information about the Corporate Golf Day and other fundraising events ......

Be invited to Scientific Retreats ......

Receive information about arranging a bequest ......

Support the Foundation in other ways ......

Please accept my / our total payment of $................

Cheques/Money Orders payable to: The CY O'Connor ERADE Village Foundation.
OR
Please debit my **Credit Card** with the above total amount only. I understand that American Express, Diners, Mastercard or VISA are accepted. My card details are as follows:

Card Type: ....

Card No.: .... Expiry Date ...../.....

Cardholder's Name: .... Signature ....

POST TO: THE C. Y. O'CONNOR ERADE VILAGE FOUNDATION INC.
PO BOX 5100 CANNING VALE SOUTH WA 6155

AL & M DAWKINS FOUNDATION

Sponsors up to

$200,000 p.a. for Research & Development in WA

Residential scholarships and grants for:

FUTURE OF WA BIOMEDICAL RESEARCH

In association with a university within WA if enrolled. Matching funding must be available or anticipated.
Expressions of interest including track record should be addressed to:

CY O'Connor Village,
PO Box 5100, Canning Vale 6155

Closing Date

November 30th or May 31st each year

The AL & M Dawkins Foundation has been funded to support problem solving in Western Australia by:

(1) Defining important issues relating to urban development and planning potential solutions thereto;
(2) Defining important issues relating to biomedical research and solutions thereto;
(3) Supporting prospective innovators in the above fields and by funding awards, scholarships, prizes and fellowships in association with CY O'Connor ERADE Village, or any branches thereof, in association with any university to which the CY O'Connor ERADE Village may be associated;
(4) Provide funding for patent costs to protect any intellectual property developed.

Applications received by November 30 or May 31 each year will be evaluated by one of two expert panels which make recommendations to the Advisory Board.

The Board ay seek further advice and will also consider:

(1) the relevance to multidisciplinary projects underway within the CYO
(2) the value of the individual to life within the village
(3) the capacity to leverage other funds
(4) university linkages
(5) potential IP

And will offer funding and accommodation for live-in researchers.

The town planning panel will be seeking to support innovative projects relating to water shortages and contamination, affordable housing, sustainable villages and isolated communities.

The biomedical panel will identify boutique projects which can be internationally competitive whilst relevant to local issues such as DNA matching, evolutionary genetics, livestock diseases and plant genomics.

Within 3 months, the administrators of the fund will advise applicants in the following categories

(1) successful
(2) for reconsideration when matching funding is confirmed
(3) invitation to reapply in the next cycle
(4) unsuccessful

Grants, generally of $50,000 must include a stipend and rental but ma also include funds for technical support, equipment, reagents, patents and publications. Travel grants will not be considered. The Foundation may decide to make no awards. Funds will only be released after assignment of IP in return for a royalty negotiated on a case by case basis.

Table of Contents

Board of Management

as of April 2017

Appointed Members

Professor Roger L. Dawkins - Research Director/Chairman
MD, DSc, FRACP, FRCPA, FRCP
Mr. Anthony Lloyd - Vice Chairman
BSc (Agric.) (Hons), MBA, LLB
Mr. Alan Peggs, - Deputy Chairman
B.Ec, M. Sc (Agric.), B.A. Hons
Mr. Renny Lee-Steere - Deputy Vice Chairman
EMBA
Mr. Ben Dawkins - Honorary Secretary
LLB
Mr. Aaron LoCicero - Deputy Honorary Secretary

Mr. Wayne Cox - Honorary Treasurer
MTax, DipFS(FP), CPA
Mr. Jason Wallis -Deputy Honorary Treasurer
(BBus, R.E.Lic)

Elected Members

Mr. Rob Giura
Mr. Richard Harper
Mr. Brian Walker
Vacant

Co-opted Members (by Invitation)

Dr. Sally Lloyd (BSc, PhD)
Mr. Dom Bayard
Dr. Sam T Dawkins

Life Members

Dr. BJ Stewart, BVSc (Hons), Dip Ag
Mr. John Heydon, BCom, CA, FTIA
Mr. Lindsay Wolridge
Dr. Edward J Steele
Ms. Sue Lester

Patron

Mr. S.L. Perron AM

Vice-Patrons

The Hon. Kim Beazley MA, MPhil
Mr. John Garland
Mr. Patrick Dawkins
Mr. Syd Martin

Executive Reports

Chairman's Report

Professor Roger Dawkins

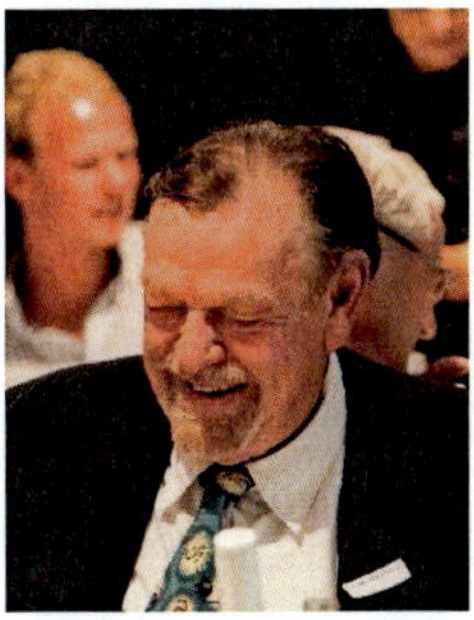

Feature Interview by Future Directions International

Local in Solution but International in Benefit

1. WHAT IS THE BASIS OF YOUR RESEARCH AND STUDENT INVOLVEMENT?

The key is the multidisciplinary MURDOCH UNIVERSITY CYO CONNOR CENTRE FOR INNOVATION IN AGRICULTURE which is developing the capacity to address and hopefully solve some of problems confronting landowners, farmers, local authorities and residents in the Peel region.

The issues have been clear for decades but remain largely intractable. We think it is time to recognise that solutions should be locally driven.

Pragmatism teaches that precious ideas and skills can be provided with opportunities through collaboration, hard-earned credibility and thence scale. We know that there are many highly skilled farmers able to teach but with no students. Unfortunately, there are many younger folks seeking some form of education or training but without any particular relevance to the problems requiring solution.

Connecting the teachers to students is a challenge. One approach is to encourage the enjoyment of problem solving. This actually means developing comparative trials designed to produce significant results capable of yielding substantial reproducible conclusions. By contrast, we hear many advocates of some product, invention or procedure promising some outcome but rarely is there a capacity to convince others as is required to be credible, to improve practices and to adapt to ever increasing challenges. Many of the enthusiasts become dispirited cranks.

Sometimes, it is as simple as knowing how to learn what has been done already and how to develop a critical capacity beyond that found in the media or a search engine. Other times, it is just a matter of very simple experimental design, such as the number of informative replicates

2. WHAT IS DRIVING YOU TOWARDS SUCH AN ACHIEVEMENT?

The relocation of the C Y O'CONNOR ERADE VILLAGE to North Dandalup provides skills, facilities and funding to support problem solving in the Peel region. The lessons from the earlier success include:

- Multidisciplinary interaction,
- Live-in incubators
- Regular but informal meetings of teachers, students and visiting experts
- Access to workshops, laboratories and computing,
- Management of intellectual property
- Quarterly retreats for assessment and planning
- Collaboration with Murdoch University
- Soft entry through activities which might engage troublesome but potentially useful youth

Now, we will add access to working farms, rural life style and commercial shopfronts so that success can translate to start-ups and financial success including, hopefully, for the otherwise unemployable.
The village should continue to create enjoyment through collaboration.

3. HOW WILL YOU ACHIEVE THESE OUTCOMES? What capabilities do you already have in place and what new capabilities will you need to develop?

Through the collaborative agreement between CYOEVF, TMG and MU, we already have basic facilities including the Dairy LAB and the ALMDF centre. Projects will drive further growth.
Examples include:

Improved pasture and reduced nutrient contamination of estuaries.

The coastal plain, as illustrated by John Peel's experience, is not naturally productive but has become so through adaptation of practices. Sand deficient in trace elements is now highly valued but is threatened because the necessary fertilizers are said to be polluting the estuaries. Fortunately, pastures have adapted and can now access the abundant superficial water with its nutrients. Which pastures and how? These questions cannot be answered on the web. The laboratory will need to be able to measure the components and identify the different varieties.

Healthy food

Unfortunately, there is very little science in the common perception of healthy food. We have selected one measurable: low melting temperature (Tm) fat, mainly because it can be measured more accurately than marketing terms like organic, pure or friendly. So we measure Tm and can provide results for local producers.

Soil health

Farmers need pertinent results rather than soil testing which is the much the same year upon year and of very little value. Our ambition is to apply a treatment to one area and to compare to another with a different treatment

Widespread use of DNA testing for food security.

Food fraud is a challenge because the food producers seem to be less nimble than the retailers. In the domestic beef market, TMG has found that approximately 25% of product is replaced or "substituted" with another which is always inferior with respect to healthiness. In export markets, the figure is much higher. CYOEVF has a simple solution based on cheap DNA testing at stages along the supply chain.

4. DO YOU SEE YOURSELF BECOMING INVOLVED WITH A PARTNER AND HOW WILL THIS WORK?

We would be very pleased to grow the partnership with FDI. We have engaged with the Chair and CEO and have offered to arrange some formal trials designed to improve soil health in this particularly interesting part of the world. Regenerative farming practices have been applied by many of our

collaborators but there is still much to do.
For example, as explained above, Kikuyu is changing and adapting. Now, the roots can be encouraged to access the superficial aquifer and strip out contained nutrients. The microbial environment is also adapting. So as to optimise these changes, we propose to develop comparative grazing zones which will allow formal testing of the many hypotheses discussed at our meetings. To this end we are collaborating with local industries such as GREENACRES, MZI and C-wise. Our challenge is to provide laboratory services which will allow farmers to draw conclusions whilst also providing these companies with valuable Intellectual Property, some of problems to be solved include

- What types of soil amendment?
- How much irrigation and when?
- Which varieties of Kikuyu and which synergistic nitrogen fixing legumes?
- Which trace elements and how to deal with heavy metal contaminants?

We see a three way mutually beneficial partnership between FDI, Murdoch University and CYOEVF. We plan to encourage the younger farmers to address these issues whilst enrolled for a degree. In this way they can enjoy the discipline and benefits of formal study whilst they solve these practical and commercial important problems.

Existing partnerships now extend well beyond Peel and WA. CYOEVF has established a laboratory in Victoria mainly for the purposes of providing breeders nationally with cost-effective DNA testing. We are now doing the same in Texas USA.

5. WHO WILL BENEFIT FROM YOUR PROPOSAL AND WHAT DO YOU CONSIDER THESE BENEFITS MIGHT BE?

The CIA of Murdoch University is unashamedly parochial in that the aim is to solve local problems on a continuing basis. It is clear that we will have a full agenda dealing with all the challenges as a consequence of increasing

- demand for healthy food,
- food fraud,

- activism from fringe groups
- threats to near urban agriculture,

but we are confident that many of the solutions will translate world-wide. So, we adopt the optimistic credo:

Local in Solution but International in Benefit.

History of the Peel region

The earliest known inhabitants of the Peel were Aborigines of the Pindjarup dialect group of the Noongar people. At the time of the first European settlement in the area in 1830, this community of Aborigines was thought to have numbered around 100. They lived in three main groups near the Murray River and along the coastal plain.

Under the program known as the Peel Settlement Scheme, organised by Thomas Peel,the initial European settlement of the Peel began shortly after the establishment of the Swan River Colony in 1829. Settlers migrated to land along the coast between Armadale and the Murray River.

Poor administration and inadequate supplies saw many of the original settlers perish through malnutrition within the first few months. The remaining settlers dispersed and a number ventured inland towards Pinjarra, where the fertile soils and grassy plains offered better opportunities for cropping and cattle grazing.

In 1846 a lead, silver and zinc mine was established at Yarrabah (near what is now Mundijong townsite). Although the mine closed the following year, due to the shaft being flooded, it re-opened on a number occasions over the next 60 years. The site is generally recognised as Western Australia's first mining operation.

Agriculture and forestry continued to be the dominant economic activity in the Peel during those early years. Whilst prime agricultural inland areas were developed, growth was restricted on the coastal plain areas due to poor drainage. This issue was finally addressed in the 1920s with the construction of a man-made drainage network that increased the amount of arable land available for development.

The Jarrahdale timber mill was commissioned in May 1872 and became the State's largest timber operation. Later that year the Rockingham-Jarrahdale railway line was completed to transport timber to the coast for use around the State and for export overseas. The durability of the timber resulted in jarrah blocks being used for paving the streets of London and Glasgow during the 1890s.

The construction of the Perth-Picton railway, along the base of the Darling Range, in 1893 led to the development of inland settlements such as Mundijong, Waroona and Dwellingup. These towns were to become service centres for the developing timber industry.

Boddington - named after an early settler - was established in 1912 and services an area of broadacre mixed wheat-sheep farming. The following year the settlement of Byford was established as a workers' housing estate, following the establishment of a major brickworks.

In 1930 dairying began to emerge as a major economic activity in the Waroona area, and this was further enhanced in 1932, when Nestles established a factory in the town to process dairy products.

Since the 1970s, resource development has had a major impact on the growth of the Peel region. In particular, the establishment of alumina refineries near Pinjarra and Wagerup, and goldmines at Boddington, have provided a considerable boost to the local population and economy. The City of Mandurah, whilst benefiting indirectly from these mining operations, continues to enjoy tremendous growth, based primarily on tourism, commerce and retail activities.

(Sourced from mandurahwa.com downloaded 13/06/2018)

Map of early Peel Settlement

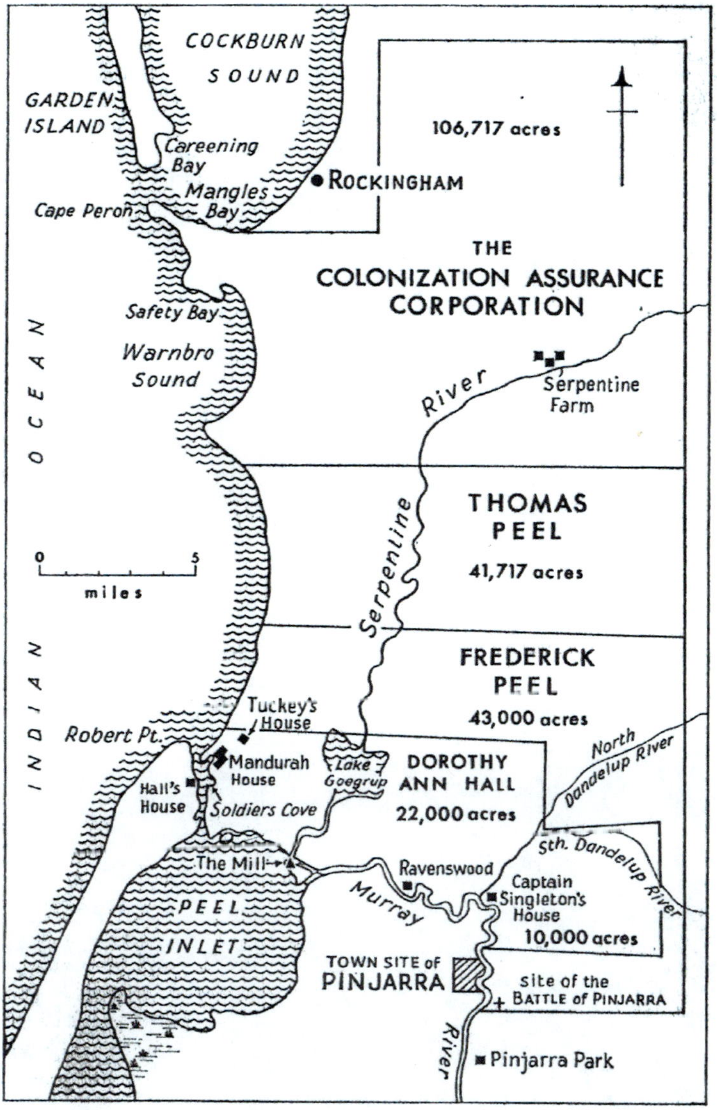

Fig. 12. Sketch map showing the partition of the Cockburn Sound Location

R

From: Thomas Peel of Swan River, Alexandra Hasluck, Oxford University Press, Melbourne, 1965

Deputy Research Director's Report

Dr Sally S Lloyd

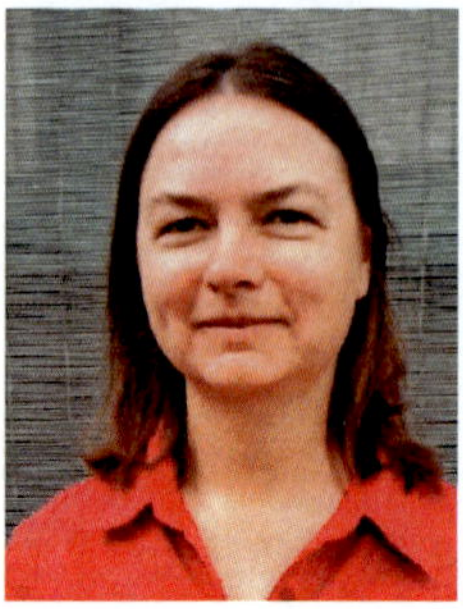

Staff and Students

The CYO laboratory welcomed two new technical staff in 2017, Matthew Nippierd and Joanne Rollinson. Both have previous experience in chemical laboratories and have quickly picked up CYO methods in DNA extraction and PCR. Jose Valenzuela, who has been working with CYO and Melaleuka Stud became formally enrolled with Murdoch University and took up a CYO PhD scholarship. John Blinco joins CYO in 2018.

Publications

In 2017 two papers with the results of two years of CYO testing of the relationship between Tm, cattle breeds, feeding and breed specific haplotypes of Chromosome 19.

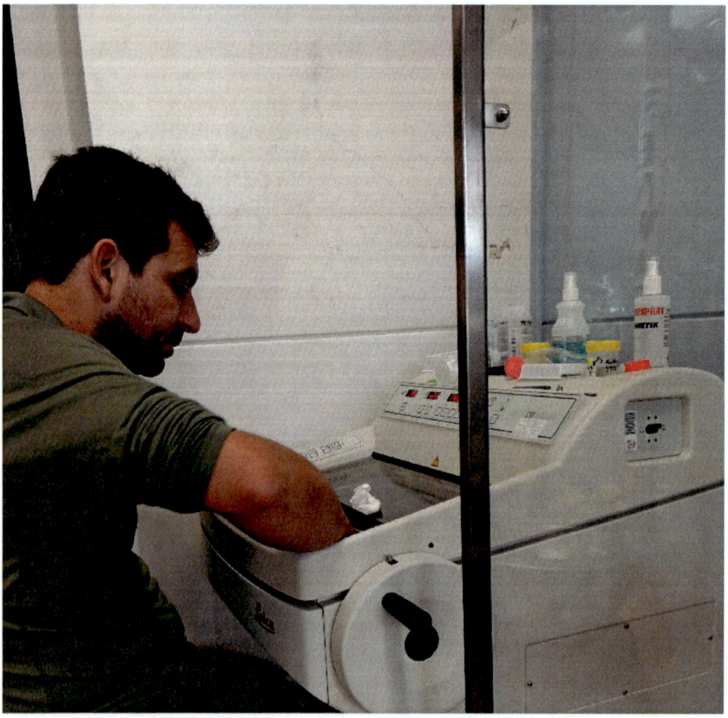

Jose Valenzuela cuts frozen sections of marbled muscle using the Cryostat at Murdoch University

Grants

Tony Lloyd was successful in obtaining a grant to research kikuyu improvement under the Royalties for Regions, Peel Regional Grants Scheme. In 2017 samples were collected from across south western WA, and also interstate and classified into genetic groups using CYO's patented BACD test. This work will continue in 2018 identifying the differences in growth and feed quality characteristics and linking them to the genetic differences found with BACD testing.

Current Research projects

In March of 2017 CYO, in collaboration with Melaleuka Stud and Milne Feed, started a trial comparing the effect of different feed formulations on growth, marbling and Tm of cattle. This research uses animals paired for similar genetics, and previous growth rates, a technique borrowed from clinical trials in human health. Pairing removes much of the genetic variability and gives statistically significant results with smaller trials. It also allows the trials to fit within Melaluka Stud's continuous production system. The results will be published in 2018 and form part of Jose Valenzuela's PhD research.

Success with this initial feed trial demonstrates the usefulness

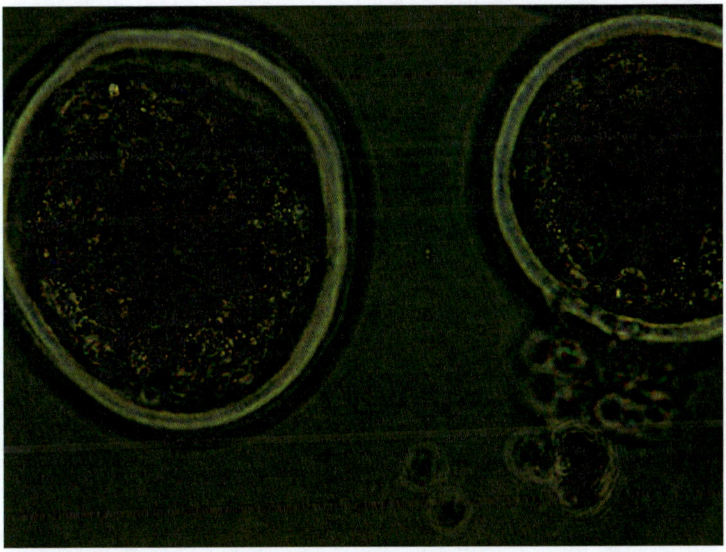

These embryos were cut in half under the microscope and implanted in different cows to produce identical twins for future feed trials

of the paring technique. In 2018 we will apply the same pairing technique to compare other feed systems, including different pasture types and including pairing based on breed specific haplotypes.

Feed trials with identical twins would allow complete elimination of the genetic variation. To this end we asked Dom Bayard to visit in October and produce a set of split embryos flushed from Melalueka Red Wagyu and implanted into Recipient Dams in Melaleuka's commercial herd. The twin calves produced from this exercise will be invaluable for future research into the effects of feed and production regimes.

The main aim of CYO research into beef is to understand the complex interaction between genetics, feeding and the production of highly marbled beef with low Tm fat. It has become clear that we need to examine the marbling at a microscopic level and to track these changes over time. Jose Valenzuela is developing techniques to take sequential biopsies of animals with varying genetics, developing

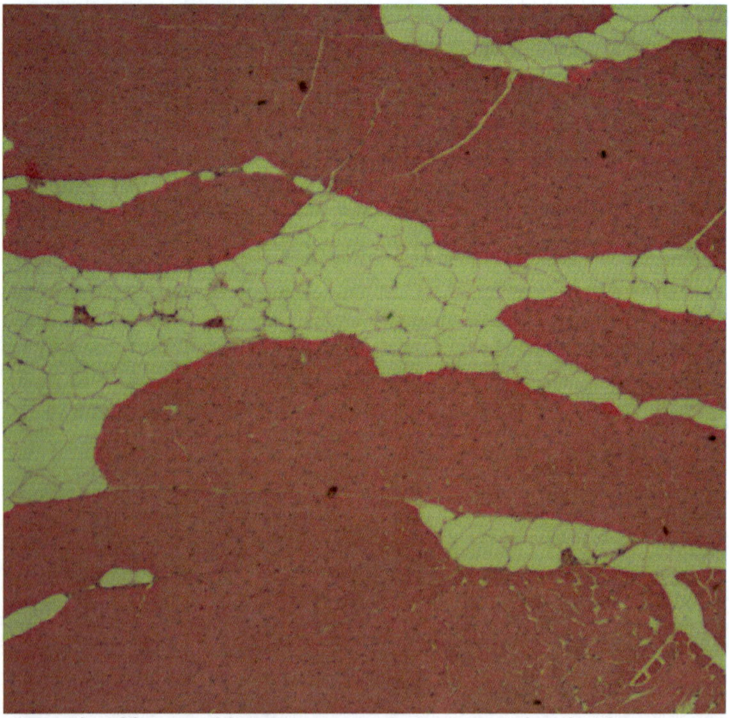

Example of fine marbling pattern at a microscopic level. Adipocytes form patterns of arborisation from around neurovascular bundles and extend along the fascicle boundaries.

marbling under various feeding strategies. Results so far have produced fascinating patterns of adipogenesis illuminated by histological examination of samples taken from the carcass. Results so far show good correlation between fat type and distribution of the tail and loin muscles. This will open the possibility for studying the changes in marbling over time by taking sequential biopsies of muscle and fat tissue.

New facilities.

With a substantial increase in activity, personnel and variety of techniques the temporary laboratory set up within Melaleuka Stud is bursting at the seams. We are looking forward to expanding into the new facilities within North Dandalup town in 2018.

Patents

Patent for the "Methods of Genotyping Livestock" patent in Europe was granted in August 2017. We chose to validate the application in the UK, France, Germany, Ireland, Switzerland and Sweden. This patent is also accepted in Australia, Japan and USA.

National Phase Patent applications for "Methods and Systems for Measuring Melting Temperatures" have been submitted in Australia and the United States.

Vice-Chairman's Report — Mr. Anthony Lloyd

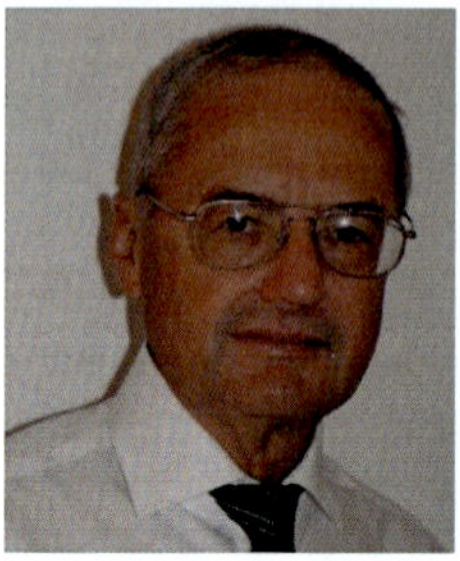

The Cargill/Branhaven Patent Litigation

During 2017 Meat and Livestock Australia and Dairy Australia brought an appeal in the Federal Court against the granting of a patent to Cargill Inc and Branhaven LLC (both United States entities) relating to the cattle genome.

The patent in issue was titled "Compositions, methods and systems for inferring bovine traits". It had been first filed in the United States in 2002 and this appeal related to the application in Australia dating from 2003.

The MLA and Dairy Australia was concerned that the granting of this patent would mean that research in Australia into bovine genetics would be seriously inhibited because the benefit of such research would be captured by the patent-holders, to the detriment of the Beef and Dairy industry.

Over the last ten years, bovine genetics has been a focus of the Foundation's research program and we have had granted a patent in Australia and the United States in relation to a part of the bovine genome. For these reasons we took a close interest in this litigation.

To understand the issues involved, it is necessary to summarize the science and technology underlying the Cargill/Branhaven patent.

SNP technology

Across the bovine genome (like all plant and animal genomes) are numerous locations where a single nucleotide is different between individuals (i.e. polymorphic) but on either side of that location there are no differences between individuals. These locations are called "single nucleotide polymorphisms" or SNPs.

Researchers identify SNPs locations more or less randomly distributed across the genome and which each has a reasonable level of variation within the population. It is then possible to obtain, for an individual, at each of these selected locations, the actual nucleotide (A, C, G or T). Of course, for each location an individual will have two outcomes, corresponding to each of its pair of chromosomes.

The technology has developed to a point where very large numbers of SNPs can be encoded onto a silicon chip and the selected SNP profile for an individual to be produced very cheaply for each individual. The current technology commercially in use in the beef and cattle industry has 70,000 SNPs and the cost to produce a profile is just a few dollars for each individual.

Of course, the challenge has been to link the SNP profile to phenotype outcomes. The process of identifying SNPs tells us nothing about the effect (if any) of a particular polymorphism either at the molecular level or at the phenotype level.

No doubt there are some SNPs which directly cause variation in the individual phenotype but it has been thought that the importance of a polymorphism is likely to be the association with other nearby polymorphisms which have a direct effect.

The development of the SNP technology has spawned numerous studies across many species to identify statistical associations between the SNP profile and an individual's phenotype.

The Cargill/Branhaven Patent

In 2002, the SNP technology was at a very early stage. The researchers responsible for the patent application identified only approximately 2,500 SNPs across the bovine genome. They had very little information as to associations between that SNP profile and economically important traits but they were able to present these as a *method* to identify individual animals with superior traits for breeding or other purposes. They also claimed that due to the well established tendency for sequences close together to be inherited together, to claim not only the method based on the original panel of 2,500 SNPs but also any panel containing SNPs within 500,000 nucleotides either side of those original 2,500 SNPs. By this device, the patent had effective coverage of an estimated 60% of the bovine genome!

The Course of the Litigation

The MLA's appeal in the Federal Court was argued in May, June and July 2017 and Justice Beach's decision was delivered on 9 February 2018 in a 260 page judgement.

The MLA had argued against the granting of the Cargill/Branhaven patent on a wide range of grounds. The judge held that as a "method" patent there was no basis of the MLA's argument that the subject matter of the patent was not patentable. He also held that the patent was "novel" and that there was a clear "inventive step".

Justice Beach did, however, accept the MLA's arguments that the patent lacked clarity and definition in certain aspects. He was concerned that the level of association between a trait and two or more SNPs would need to be established and suggested a statistical test of significance (p=0.01). He was also concerned that the region on either side of the identified SNPs where additional SNPs could be identified within the patent should be subject to a test of linkage disequilibrium. Branhaven was allowed time to amend their patent application to address these concerns.

At the time of writing the issue of amendment to the patent application has not been resolved.

Comments

If Branhaven is permitted to amend their patent application within the terms of Justice Beach's concerns there would not be much practical effect on the breadth of the Cargill/Branhaven patent. Any economically important association between SNPs and a trait should be able to be established with the required level of statistical significance.

The case for including the 500,000 nucleotide sequence each side of the nominated SNPs within the patent coverage is based on expected levels of linkage disequilibrium across the genome so it is only in the case of recombination "hotspots" where addressing the judge's concerns will have a practical effect on the breadth of the Cargill/Branhaven patent. These are likely limited in number.

While the litigation is not finally resolved (and there may, in any case, be further appeals) the case underlines the opportunity for very broad "method" patents to be granted at early stages in the emergence of new technologies and their application to new fields.

Despite the substantial legal success of the owners of the Cargill/Branhaven patent (to date) there remain substantial questions as to the value of the SNP technology to the breeding and selection of livestock. In many of the published studies the association between SNPs and production characteristics are weak. Claims for successful application of the technology are often obscured by the proponents' failure to publish their results in a verifiable form. The economic value of the patent is also fast eroding with a record date of 2002.

There are also good scientific reasons to expect that the SNP approach which forms the basis of the Branhaven patent will rarely form the basis of identifying strong associations between phenotype and genotype in livestock.

The CYOEVF Patent

The researchers at the Foundation have adopted a different approach to the identification of superior genetics in livestock, based on the identification of Ancestral Haplotypes as a source of genetic variation within a species.

The Foundation's research group played a major role in establishing that many of the richly polymorphic regions in the human genome (therefore the regions which are the source of much of the genetic variation within the species) are regions which are inherited unchanged from generation to generation (i.e. they are regions within areas where recombination is suppressed). Applying this insight to the cattle genome, the research group identified a 4 Mb region on Chromosome 19 which contained many of the genes responsible for the regulation of muscle growth, fat deposition and desaturation of saturated fat, which is richly polymorphic but highly conserved.

The identification of the different haplotypes within the C19 region, the variation of haplotype frequency between cattle breeds and the association between these haplotypes and the economically important traits such as intramuscular fat composition, marbling, intramuscular fat melting point and muscle growth was the basis of the Foundation's patent "Methods of Genotyping Livestock" granted in 2015 in the United States and in Australia in 2016.

While the Foundation's patent covers only part of one chromosome, it is clearly an important region for meat quality. The patent also extends to all livestock including goats, sheep and pigs.

With the Foundation's patent having a record date of 2009 the Foundation's and it has been granted without challenge in both the United States in Australia, there is a strong basis of developing and commercializing this aspect of the Foundation's research program.

Deputy Vice Chairman — Mr Renny Lee-Steere

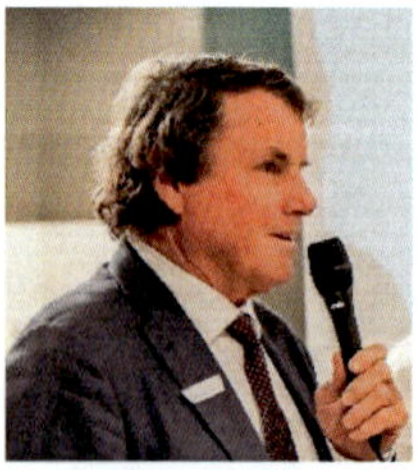

South West Livestock Producers Facing Another Sub Clover Crisis.

The majority of Livestock producers throughout the Avon Valley, west to Williams and south to Mt Barker and Esperance were faced with a crisis during the winter and spring of 2017 when it became apparent that their sub clover pastures were being wiped out and now with summer rainfall events through the first months of 2018 they may be facing a repetition for the coming winter and spring.

This unwelcome occurrence was identified as Sub Clover Red Leaf Virus (SCRLV). This phenomenon has been reported to occur in Esperance region for a number of years, however, following the dry winter in much of the south west of WA in 2017, sub clover leaves were turning red and eventually dying.

The source of the virus has been identified as Soya Bean Dwarf Virus, a luteovirus, which needs a constant green host for survival and spreads by Aphids which once they become infectious can spread the virus for the rest of their life.

Symptoms of SCRLV on Sub Clover include, intense reddening of the older leaves starting at the leaf margins before spreading across the whole leaf. Infected plants are stunted, and many fail to set seed. The spread across a paddock can be very quick and by the time a farmer sees symptoms, (around 3 weeks from infection), it is too late to do anything.

Fertiliser application (phosphorous, potash or nitrogen) does not alleviate virus symptoms. Spraying aphids can be uneconomic, unless you are able to identify the presence of aphids at a very early stage.

Only virus testing can confirm the presence of SCRLV. Fresh clover plants can be submitted to the WA Agricultural Dept Laboratory Services- Plant Pathology team to be tested and confirmed if it is present or not.

To better understand the spread and extent of the syndrome, Meat and Livestock Australia (MLA) and Australian Wool Innovation (AWI) have developed a survey to enable producer to share their experiences. MLA and AWI are planning to bring together a cross disciplinary group of researchers, pasture agronomists, and extension experts to assist producers in how to best manage their pasture.

Sub Clover are widespread throughout South Western Australia, with around 13 million hectares of pastures that are mostly sub clover. While MLA and AWI over many years have invested in legumes such as Serradella and Bisarrula which are not affected by SCRLV, the organisations acknowledge the sub clover is an important basis for any pasture system and without functioning legumes, pastures significantly loose productivity and cannot sustain current livestock production. At a time when livestock production is riding high, with excellent farmgate prices, it will be a disaster

if pastures failed our producers.
Renny Lee-Steere
"Hawthornden"
Toodyay

Honorary Secretary — Mr Ben Dawkins

During 2017 the administration of the Foundation went down an entirely new path. September 11th was the 'go live' date for the staff of the Centre for Innovation in Agriculture becoming Murdoch Employees. This has resulted in reasonably streamlined administration in so far as the payment of staff is concerned, with Murdoch University invoicing the Foundation quarterly to recover wages paid to the employees. Murdoch pays the on-costs and some superannuation for the staff and it is hoped that as more projects take hold and more students are enrolled, the Murdoch contribution will increase and will help the Centre to become even more collaborative.

The structure of the Centre for Innovation in Agriculture needs to be fully populated with the addition of at least one administrator and one or more Academics (Research Fellows) at Level B and above. This will allow more projects and students to be taken on and more exciting contributions to be made by the Centre. The commitment to the Centre is undoubted, with a 10 year pipeline of funding being committed by the Foundation.

Other governance issues are being managed very well. For example the changes effected by the Incorporated Associations Act 2015 (WA) have resulted in necessary improvements to the way governance issues are documented in our minutes and also in some changes to our reporting. Several of these have been implemented already with the final change to be a redrafting of our constitution prior 1 July 2019 as required by the new Act. Significantly, the Australian Charities and Not for Profits Commission now recognises the Foundation as having the following four charitable aims (increased from three previously); Advancing Education, Promotion, Prevention and Control of Diseases in Humans, Advancing Health and A Purpose Beneficial to the General Public (Specifically, Advancement of Agriculture).

In 2018, I foresee significant growth for the activities of the Foundation at the North Dandalup Centre. This will be affected to some extent by funding applications. The Piara Waters incubators are fully tenanted and ready for subdivision and sale which will provide a further injection of funds, quite likely during the latter part of 2018. The success at Piara Waters will no doubt be built upon at North Dandalup by focusing on multi-disciplinary collaboration and supporting inventors and those who wish to commercialise their research, including research conducted as part of their PhD. This was behind the success of the Piara Waters site and will be followed closely as the North Dandalup site develops. Education, Research and Development and Employment, 'ERADE' remains the focus at North Dandalup with the addition of 'Innovation' as reflected in the name of the new Centre.

Honorary Treasurer's Report — Mr. Wayne Cox

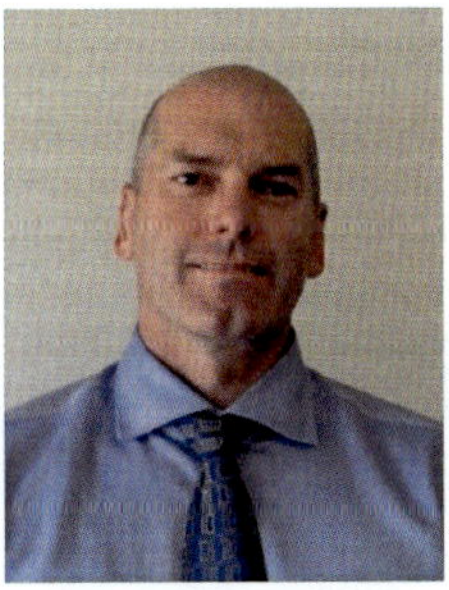

I am pleased to report that the Foundation is in its strongest financial position for years.

We have 1.3M in the term deposits and an operating cash flow surplus of $94,909.00. We have also been gradually selling down our GTG Shares to bolster our cash reserves.

Our rent received for the financial year from the Incubator's is the highest it has ever been at $217,480.00.

During the year we have relocated our operations to North Dandalup with a new laboratory and facilities. We are very honoured and privileged to have the support of the AL & M Dawkins Foundation who have provided the new facility and the renovation of the laboratory to the value of 1.0M.

This move now leaves the Foundation in a very strong position with our major asset in the Incubators being able to be liquidated. We expect the Incubators to be realized for approximately 7.0M in today's market with strong interest being shown already.

CYO Foundation Members Profiles

Mr. Paul Fitzpatrick

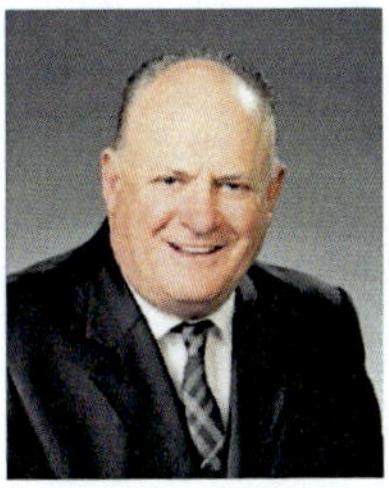

I recently joined the CY O'Connor Foundation Centre for Innovation in Agriculture to oversee their Agri-innovation incubator program for the Peel region at North Dandalup following the completion of my term as Chairman of the Peel Development Commission.

As a descendant of a pioneering Peel region family from 1893 I returned to my grassroots in 2000. From a diverse career involving an innovative internationally award winning technology company that developed the smart house concept my main focus and interest was in diversification and sustainability of the land as a research and development smart farm/lifestyle Olive grower in Waroona. My community involvement continued as a Shire President of Waroona to the appointment by the Minister for Regional Development as Chairman of the Peel Development Commission. This role emphasized my passion for the region in the formulation and work into the Peel Regional Investment Blueprint to 2050. A strategy that recognised the potential for intensive agriculture enterprises to exploit the regions proximity to large markets. A plan that has been instrumental and invaluable to the implementation of the Transform Peel project for the Peel region that has identified a 42,000 hectare Peel Food Zone, a 1,000 hectare Peel Business Park; and the Peel Integrated Water Initiative. The Transform Peel initiative will realise the vision for the Peel to be a progressive, prosperous and dynamic region that will create some 33,000 jobs over this period.

The Transform Peel project through the numerous stakeholders in the Peel region introduced me to the vision of the CY O'Connor Foundation and the Centre for Innovation in Agriculture at North Dandalup. I recognised that high quality research is necessary if the strategy was to succeed.

I am now continuing this vison for the region with the Centre of Innovation in particular with the incubator program that will see technology and diversity in the development of aspiring innovators and entrepreneurs within agriculture.

Locally involved industry include Alcoa, MZI, Eco-

Diagnostics, CarbonFix Nu-Soil, Greenacres Turf Farm and C-Wise.

Areas of interest received have been for improved pasture and reduced nutrient contamination of estuaries, traceability of meat, drone technology addressing disease crops, dung beetles, healthy nutria-food, soil health and the use of DNA testing for food security.

The land rehabilitation program with the Centre for Innovation in Agriculture for the mining industry is also seen as a positive incubator in addressing solutions for best use of farmlands for soil and water in post mining activities.

An example is Alcoa that has introduced some of the issues pertaining to mine rehabilitation and the use of the overburden known as RED MUD. As a consequence we are investigating new approaches encouraged by the need for improved agriculture. In a workshop setting we ask whether trials of new approaches could be compared.

MZI and C-Wise have been conducting trials for the rehabilitation of land use and the centre will be working with them.

Greenacres Turf Farm have been working with the centre during the Kikuyu grass research project and will continue this during the process and the overall areas of soil and water research.

An Advisory Board of Governance has been established which I chair with membership comprising of Future Directions International Major General John Hartley AO, (Retrd) CEO and renowned agriculture advisor Alan Peggs.

This board responsibilities are:

- To assist CYOEVF in establishing effective relationships with community, professional educational and government bodies
- Defining priorities in research and development
- Creating future funding for projects, incubators, infrastructure and staffing.

In March Major General Michael Jeffery (Retd) who chairs the Soils for Life program established by the Federal Government in 2012 visited the centre. The Soils for Life program are very keen to establish a trial at the Centre for Innovation in Agriculture at North Dandalup.

I see the Centre for Innovation in Agriculture as a priority in today's world. Traditional farmers only get 40 attempts (seasons) at farming in their lifetime from there 20's to 60's. The Centre for Innovation at North Dandalup with the incubator program gives innovators/entrepreneurs numerous attempts each year.

The Centre for Innovation will ensure we have a healthy food bowl, soil and water management with high quality research and development for all Western Australians.

The CY O'Connor Foundation Charity Golf Day held at the Mandurah Country Club

The annual C.Y. O'Connor ERADE Village Foundation Charity Golf Day was held on the 11 May at the WA Golf Industry 2017 Metropolitan Facility of the Year Mandurah Country Club.

This year we had a record number of corporate and supporters

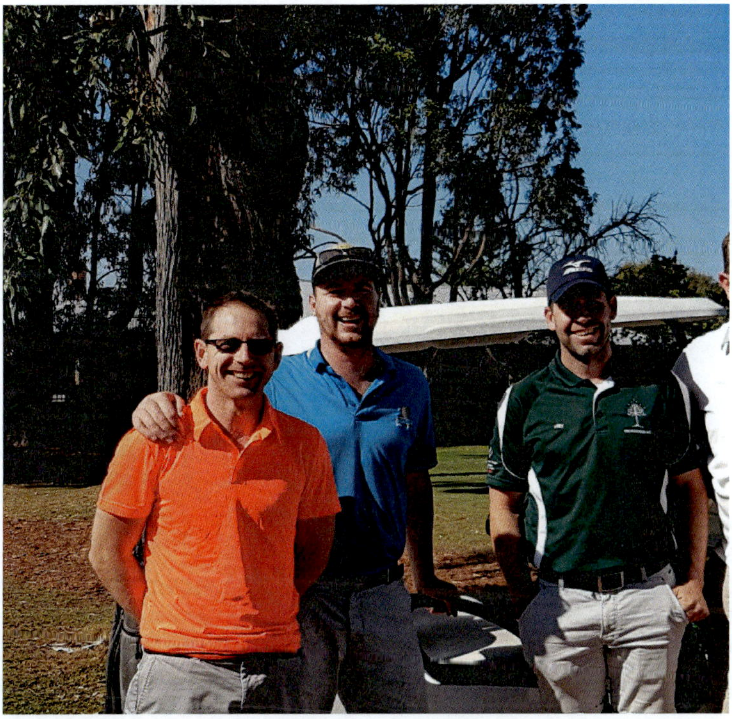

Teams get ready for a day of golf at Mandurah Country Club. From left to right: Steven Smith, Nat Broomfield, Brad Hill and Ben Dawkins.

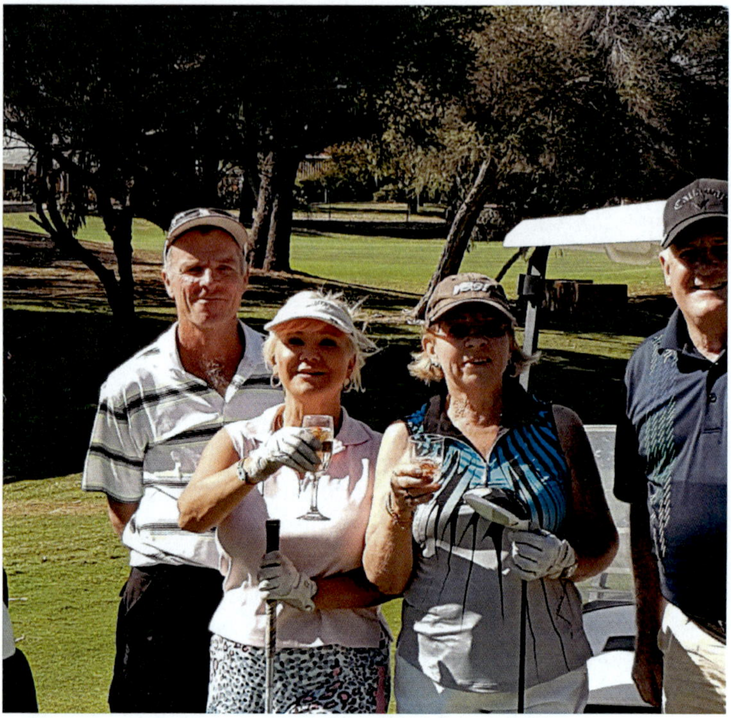

Winners of the golf day. From left to right: Brendan Corver, Eleni Fitzpatrick, Anita English and Paul Fitzpatrick.

of the foundation attending for golf and enjoying the hospitality over dinner of the Mandurah Country Club facilities in private rooms overlooking the course.

Winners on the day won the right to play in the 2018 Peel Pro AM and this year we did see a very competitive field that was won by the CarbonFix Nu-Soil Pty Ltd team of Anita English and Brendan Corver who combined with Paul and Eleni Fitzpatrick.

The golf gods were onside and provided beautiful weather for the day and our thanks go to Ben Dawkins who MC'd for the day but more importantly to our sponsors who continue to support the foundation.

Special thanks also to Grant Shortland-Jones, General Manager of the Mandurah Country Club for his assistance in preparing the day and the donation of golf games with carts for our silent auction.

Mr Dom Bayard

Report to the C Y O'Connor Foundation Board 28/3/18

CEG has had a very mixed few months in terms of laboratory output during 2018. Whilst we have continued to collect and extract DNA samples from Wagyu carcasses and tail hair samples, we have had issues with retaining quality laboratory staff due to a number of factors. This has led to very fragmented results and a lack of continuity in the lab.

We have been continuing to collect over 100 meat and fat samples monthly from fullblood Wagyu carcasses at Pakenham that have all been fed under the same conditions on the same feedlot, thus providing a very good source of research material. We have been taking camera images from these carcasses, which gives accurate data on marbling %, marbling fineness and coarseness amongst a plethora of detailed information. We have pedigree information on a large proportion of these carcasses so we are able to look at the difference between sire lines.

Figure 1: Average Fat Melting Point vs Carcass Weight

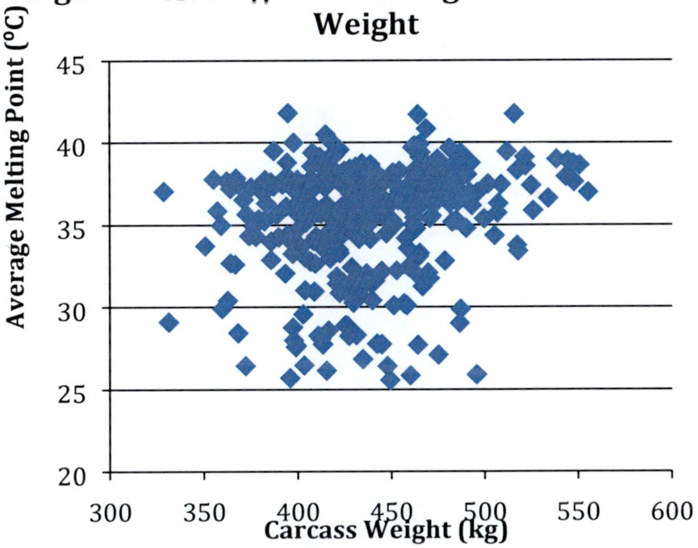

Figure 2:Average Melting point for Sires with 5+ progeny

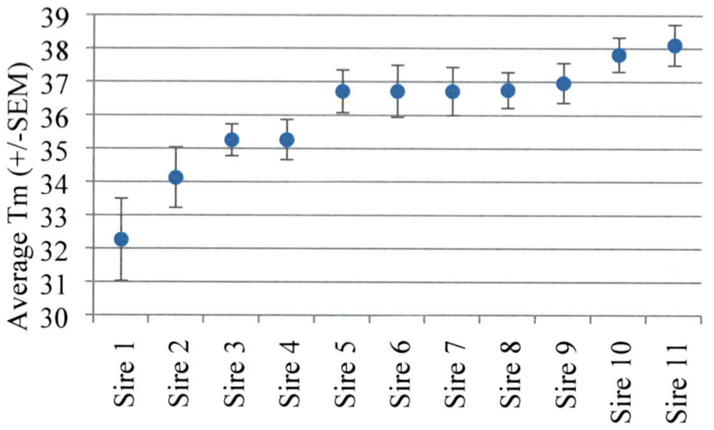

We now have nearly 500 samples collected and with carcass data on all these we are proposing to haplotype many of these in the near future when we have the resources to run them through the system.

In terms of commercial samples being submitted, I have been loath to take these on until I have a quality team in place that can assure quick turn-around times with assured quality control. Certainly, the haplotype story on marbling in Wagyu is one that can be seen in the results coming through and so I hope that I can report to the board in the near future in a much more positive light.

Financial Statements

IMMUNOGENETICS RESEARCH FOUNDATION WA INC
T/AS
THE C.Y. O'CONNOR ERADE VILLAGE FOUNDATION
67 161 830 965

FINANCIAL REPORT
FOR THE YEAR ENDED
31 December 2017

PASCOE PARTNERS ACCOUNTANTS
CERTIFIED PRACTISING ACCOUNTANTS

IMMUNOGENETICS RESEARCH FOUNDATION WA INC
T/A
THE C.Y. O'CONNOR ERADE VILLAGE FOUNDATION
67 161 830 965

CONTENTS

IMMUNOGENETICS RESEARCH FOUNDATION WA INC
T/A
THE C.Y. O'CONNOR ERADE VILLAGE FOUNDATION
67 161 830 965
C Y O'CONNOR HI-TECH INCUBATOR CENTRE
DEPARTMENTAL TRADING, PROFIT AND LOSS STATEMENT
FOR THE YEAR ENDED 31 DECEMBER 2017

	Note	2017 $	2016 $
C Y O'CONNOR HI-TECH INCUBATOR CENTRE			
OTHER INCOME			
Lease Rentals		217,480	198,980
EXPENSES			
Bad Debts Written Off	2	-	812
Cleaning		4,160	-
Depreciation - Plant & Equipment	3	2,003	2,462
Depreciation - Buildings		25,886	26,647
Electricity		9,653	
Leasing Fees		9,561	
Incubator Management Fees		6,787	15,515
Repairs & Maintenance	4	14,608	7,597
		72,658	53,033
SURPLUS (DEFICIT) FROM INCOME AND EXPENDITURE		144,822	145,947
Opening Balance 1st January 2017		1,481,115	1,335,168
Closing Balance 31st December 2017		1,625,937	1,481,115

IMMUNOGENETICS RESEARCH FOUNDATION WA INC
T/A
THE C.Y. O'CONNOR ERADE VILLAGE FOUNDATION
67 161 830 965
RESEARCH & GENERAL FUND
DEPARTMENTAL TRADING, PROFIT AND LOSS STATEMENT
FOR THE YEAR ENDED 31 DECEMBER 2017

	Note	2017 $	2016 $
RESEARCH & GENERAL			
Donations/Bequests		37,918	167,494
Fund Raising		7,279	-
Meeting Registration Fees		3,290	7,345
Membership Fees		6,818	3,866
Laundry & Gaming Machine sales		730	715
		56,035	179,420
OTHER INCOME			
Grant Income		55,000	-
Interest Received		31,707	25,913
Other Income		1	-
Reimbursements & Recoups		1,696	59
Profit / (Loss) on Sale of Non-Current Assets		-	(9,030)
		88,404	16,942
EXPENSES			
Accountancy & Audit Fees		5,482	4,500
Advertising		160	540
Bank Charges		235	88
Cleaning		1,561	2,145
Consultancy Fees		14,838	30,501
Contract Work		995	-
Computer Expense		-	28
Depreciation - Plant & Equipment	3	19,356	18,213
Bad Debts Written Off	2	-	5,530
Electricity		177	-
Fees & Permits		8,080	1,322
Freight & Cartage		1,903	279
Fund Raising Costs		1,000	-
Innovation Award		-	10,000
Insurance		10,326	10,526

Interest Paid		3	-
Licensing Fees		763	-
Meeting / Visitors / Honorarium		18,031	18,447
Consumables & Lab Supplies		36,366	9,829
Motor Vehicle Expense		-	756
Patent Fees		27,153	58,929
Postage		717	
Printing & Stationery		532	715
Repairs & Maintenance	4	482	-
Subscriptions		1,325	-
Superannuation Contributions		7,921	8,157
Telephone		-	4,075
Travelling Expenses		-	5,907

IMMUNOGENETICS RESEARCH FOUNDATION WA INC
T/A
THE C.Y. O'CONNOR ERADE VILLAGE FOUNDATION
67 161 830 965
RESEARCH & GENERAL FUND
DEPARTMENTAL TRADING, INCOME AND EXPENDITURE
FOR THE YEAR ENDED 31 DECEMBER 2017

	Note	2017 $	2016 $
Unrealised loss / (gain) on Shares		(24,033)	168,233
Wages		83,753	92,887
Waste Disposal		438	522
		217,564	452,129
SURPLUS (DEFICIT) FROM INCOME AND EXPENDITURE		(73,125)	(255,767)
Opening Balance 1st January 2017		1,113,977	1,369,744
Closing Balance 31st December 2017		1,040,852	1,113,977

IMMUNOGENETICS RESEARCH FOUNDATION WA INC
T/A
THE C.Y. O'CONNOR ERADE VILLAGE FOUNDATION
67 161 830 965
BALANCE SHEET
AS AT 31 DECEMBER 2017

	Note	2017 $	2016 $
TRUST FUNDS			
RESERVES	5	2,666,789	2,595,092
TOTAL TRUST FUNDS		2,666,789	2,595,092
Represented by:			
CURRENT ASSETS			
Cash on Hand		1	1
Petty Cash		111	111
Prepayments on Contract		42,282	-
Bankwest Chq A/c		2	-
Westpac Max 112867		7,204	25,650
Westpac Research Account 10-4752		7,207	(2,694)
Westpac Community Solutions Account 1645		3,870	19,471
Westpac Community Solution 2961		3,000	-
Term Deposits	8	1,308,020	1,245,336
Accounts Receivable		3,575	1,310
Loans - Unsecured	6	10,000	10,000
GST Payable (Refundable)		(2,885)	10,393
TOTAL CURRENT ASSETS		1,382,387	1,309,578
NON CURRENT ASSETS			
Fixed Assets			
Computer Equipment		364,971	364,971
Less: Accumulated Depreciation		(364,273)	(363,834)
		698	1,137
Motor Vehicles		13,500	13,500
Less: Accumulated Depreciation		(12,943)	(12,781)
		557	719
Office Furniture & Equipment		11,612	11,612
Less: Accumulated Depreciation		(11,183)	(11,076)
		429	536
Laboratory Equipment		561,092	552,725

Less: Accumulated Depreciation		(459,625)	(440,977)
		101,467	111,748
Incubators		55,124	55,124
Less: Accumulated Depreciation		(45,557)	(43,554)
		9,567	11,570
Incubator Buildings		1,287,625	1,287,625
Less: Accumulated Depreciation		(313,297)	(287,411)
		974,328	1,000,214
Total Fixed Assets		1,087,046	1,125,924
Investments			
Listed Shares in Public Companies	7	156,216	132,183
Patents		54,750	54,750
Total Investments		210,966	186,933

IMMUNOGENETICS RESEARCH FOUNDATION WA INC
T/A
THE C.Y. O'CONNOR ERADE VILLAGE FOUNDATION
67 161 830 965
BALANCE SHEET
AS AT 31 DECEMBER 2017

	Note	2017 $	2016 $
TOTAL NON-CURRENT ASSETS		1,298,012	1,312,857
TOTAL ASSETS		2,680,399	2,622,435
CURRENT LIABILITIES			
Trade Creditors		3,767	12,208
Incubator Bond Monies	9	7,970	7,970
Amounts Withheld	10	1,873	7,165
TOTAL CURRENT LIABILITIES		13,610	27,343
TOTAL LIABILITIES		13,610	27,343
NET ASSETS		2,666,789	2,595,092

IMMUNOGENETICS RESEARCH FOUNDATION WA INC
T/A
THE C.Y. O'CONNOR ERADE VILLAGE FOUNDATION
67 161 830 965
NOTES TO THE FINANCIAL STATEMENTS
FOR THE YEAR ENDED 31 DECEMBER 2017

1 Statement of Significant Accounting Policies

The director of the trustee company has prepared the financial statements of the trust on the basis that the trust is a non-reporting entity because there are no users dependent on general purpose financial statements. The financial statements are therefore special purpose financial statements that have been prepared in order to meet the needs of beneficiaries.

The financial statements have been prepared in accordance with the significant accounting policies disclosed below which the director has determined are appropriate to meet the needs of members. Such accounting policies are consistent with the previous period unless stated otherwise.

The financial statements have been prepared on an accruals basis and are based on historical costs unless otherwise stated in the notes. The accounting policies that have been adopted in the preparation of these statements are as follows:

Property, Plant and Equipment

Property, plant and equipment are carried at cost, independent or director's valuation. All assets, excluding freehold land and buildings are depreciated over the useful lives of the assets to the trust.

Increases in the carrying amount arising on revaluation of land and buildings are credited to a revaluation reserve in shareholders' equity. Decreases that offset previous increases of the same asset are charged against fair value reserves directly in equity; all other decreases are charged to the income statement. Each year the difference between depreciation based on the revalued carrying amount of the asset charged to the income statement and depreciation based on the asset's original cost is transferred from the revaluation reserve to retained earnings.

The carrying amount of plant and equipment is reviewed annually by directors to ensure it is not in excess of the recoverable amount from these assets. The recoverable amount is assessed on the basis of the expected net cash flows that will be received from the asset's employment and subsequent disposal. The expected net cash flows have not been discounted in determining recoverable amounts.

Property, Plant and Equipment (PPE)

Leasehold improvements and office equipment are carried at cost less, where applicable, any accumulated depreciation.

The depreciable amount of all PPE is depreciated over the useful lives of the assets to the trust commencing from the time the asset is held ready for use.

Leasehold improvements are amortised over the shorter of either the unexpired period of the lease or the estimated useful lives of the improvements.

IMMUNOGENETICS RESEARCH FOUNDATION WA INC
T/A
THE C.Y. O'CONNOR ERADE VILLAGE FOUNDATION
67 161 830 965
NOTES TO THE FINANCIAL STATEMENTS
FOR THE YEAR ENDED 31 DECEMBER 2017

		2017 $	2016 $
2	**Bad Debt Written Off**		
	Hi-Tech Incubator Centre	-	812
	Research & General Fund	-	5,530
		-	6,342
3	**Depreciation - Plant & Equipment**		
	Hi-Tech Incubator Centre	2,003	2,462
	Research & General Fund	19,356	18,213
		21,359	20,675
4	**Repairs & Maintenance**		
	Hi-Tech Incubator Centre	14,608	7,597
	Research & General Fund	482	-
		15,090	7,597
5	**RESERVES**		
	Reserves - Deficit	-	-
	7th MHC Evolution Meeting Fund	-	-
	C Y O'Connor Hi-Tech Incubator Centre	1,625,937	1,481,115
	Research & General Fund	1,040,852	1,113,977
		2,666,789	2,595,092
6	**Loans - Unsecured**		
	E J Steele	10,000	10,000
		10,000	10,000
7	**Listed Shares in Public Companies**		
	Listed Shares in Public Companies at Market Value	156,216	132,183

IMMUNOGENETICS RESEARCH FOUNDATION WA INC
T/A
THE C.Y. O'CONNOR ERADE VILLAGE FOUNDATION
67 161 830 965
NOTES TO THE FINANCIAL STATEMENTS
FOR THE YEAR ENDED 31 DECEMBER 2017

		2017 $	2016 $
8	**Term Deposits**		
	Westpac Term Deposit xxxxxx	102,650	100,000
	Westpac Term Deposit xxxxxx	65,539	64,192
	Westpac Term Deposit xxxxxx	131,913	128,071
	Westpac Term Deposit xxxxxx	103,000	100,000
	Westpac Term Deposit xxxxxx	128,384	125,000
	Westpac Term Deposit xxxxxx	102,669	99,999
	Westpac Term Deposit xxxxxx	104,176	101,685
	Westpac Term Deposit xxxxxx	131,791	102,047
	Westpac Term Deposit xxxxxx	104,706	102,557
	Westpac Term Deposit xxxxxx	100,000	130,276
	Westpac Term Deposit xxxxxx	-	27,317
	Westpac Term Deposit xxxxxx	102,331	100,000
	Westpac Term Deposit xxxxxx	100,861	64,192
	Westpac Term Deposit xxxxxx	30,000	
		1,308,020	1,245,336
9	**Incubator Bond Monies**		
	Auslanka	1,120	1,120
	Better Care Medical Centre	1,360	1,360
	Youme Clothing	450	450
	Spicy Wok	1,200	1,200
	Make Your Mark Art Cafe	1,040	1,040
	Renov8withus Pty Ltd	1,400	1,400
	Indebiti Solutions Pty Ltd	1,400	1,400
		7,970	7,970
10	**Amounts Withheld**		
	Amounts Withheld from Salary, Wages and Other Payments	-	4,424
	Employee Superannuation Payable	1,873	2,741
		1,873	7,165

Compilation Report

IMMUNOGENETICS RESEARCH FOUNDATION WA INC
T/A
THE C.Y. O'CONNOR ERADE VILLAGE FOUNDATION
67 161 830 965

We have compiled the accompanying special purpose financial statements of THE C.Y. O'CONNOR ERADE VILLAGE FOUNDATION which comprise the balance sheet as at 31 December 2017, profit and loss statement and cash flow statement for the year then ended, a summary of significant accounting policies and other explanatory notes.

The specific purpose for which these special purpose financial statements have been prepared is to provide information relating to the performance and financial position of the incorporated body that satisfies the information needs of the director.

The responsibility of the Director

The director is solely responsible for the information contained in the special purpose financial statements and has determined that the basis of accounting used is appropriate to meet their needs and for the purpose for which the financial statements were prepared.

Our responsibility

On the basis of information provided by the director, we have compiled the accompanying special purpose financial statements in accordance with the financial reporting framework described in Note 1 to the financial statements and APES 315: Compilation of Financial Information.

Our procedures use accounting expertise to collect, classify and summarise the financial information, which the director provided, into a financial report. Our procedures do not include verification or validation procedures. No audit or review has been performed and accordingly no assurance is expressed.

The special purpose financial statements were prepared exclusively for the director. We do not accept responsibility to any other person for the content of the special purpose financial statements.

Name of Firm: Pascoe Partners Accountants
Certified Practising Accountants

Name of Partner:

Wayne Michael Cox
MTax, Dip FS(FP), CPA, CTA

Address: Level 2, 100 Havelock Street
West Perth

Dated:

Auditor's Report

JOHN D PASCOE, FCPA

Certified Practising Accountant
Registered Tax Agent
Registered Company Auditor

Unit 10, 125 Alfred Road
Mount Claremont
Western Australia 6010

ABN 64 724 120 246 Fax: 08 9384 9050
Email: johnjill@westnet.com.au
Mob: 0406 380 215

5 April 2018

The Board of Directors CY O'Connor Erade Village Foundation Level 2 100 Havelock St West Perth WA 6005

Dear Chairperson

CY O'Connor Erade Village Foundation - Audit of Financial Reports

Thank you for your appointment of me auditor of the accounts and financial reports of the above.

For year ended 31 December 2017, I am pleased to confirm my acceptance of the appointment and would now like to set out my understanding of the terms of this engagement.

Review of the Financial Reports for Year Ended 31 December 2017

The financial report of a Foundation must be reviewed by an approved auditor. The auditor must give the Board a report on the financial report in the approved form within the prescribed time after the year of income to which the financial report relates.

The work undertaken by me to form an opinion is permeated by judgement, in particular regarding the nature, timing and extent of the review procedures forgathering of evidence and the drawing of conclusions based on the evidence gathered. In addition, there are inherent limitations in any review, and these include the use of testing, the inherent limitations of any internal control structure, the possibility of collusion to commit fraud, and the fact that most review evidence is persuasive rather than conclusive. As a result, my review can only provide reasonable - not absolute - assurance that the financial report is free from material misstatement.

I direct your attention to the fact that it is the Board's responsibility for the maintenance of adequate accounting records and internal controls, the safeguarding of The Foundation assets, the selection of accounting policies, the preparation of the special purpose financial report and returns, and compliance. I note the Board is responsible for providing access to all information that is relevant to the preparation of the financial report, and any additional information that may be required as part of the review. In particular, I note the Board is responsible for the implementation and operation of accounting and internal control systems that are designed to prevent and detect fraud and error.

Page 1 of 4

The review of the financial report does not relieve the Board of their responsibilities.

My review will be conducted in accordance with Australian Auditing Standards. The objective of the review is to obtain a reasonable assurance about whether the financial report as a whole is free from material mis-statement, whether due to fraud or error and to issue an review report on the financial report.

My review work involves examination, on a test basis, of evidence supporting the amounts and other disclosures in the financial report in order to form an opinion as to whether, in all material respects, the financial report is fairly stated in accordance with the accounting policies described in the notes thereto.

My review will be planned and conducted primarily to enable me to express my professional opinion as to whether the financial report complies with Australian Accounting Standards and other mandatory professional reporting requirements as adopted by the Board, but, also, so as to have reasonable expectation of detecting material misstatements arising as a result of irregularities which would have a material effect on the financial report. Unless otherwise agreed to, I assume no responsibility to design review procedures to identify matters that may be appropriate to report to you.

Report on Matters

I am required to inform you of certain uncorrected mis-statements identified during the review, and I must obtain representations from you acknowledging the uncorrected mis-statements have been brought to your attention, and that you have considered the effects of these mis-statements to be either material or immaterial individually and in aggregate to the financial report.

At the completion of the review I will prepare a report to advise you of any matters encountered during the course of the review that I believe should be brought to your attention. I am also required to form an opinion on the accounting policies adopted in preparing the financial report. Please note you should not assume that matters reported to you, or that a report that there are no matters to be communicated, indicates that there are no additional matters that you should be aware of in meeting your responsibilities.

Privacy and Quality Control

The conduct of my review in accordance with Australian Auditing Standards means that information acquired by me in the course of my review is subject to strict confidentiality requirements. I am also subject to the Privacy Act 1988 in the handling of personal information. I will not use any personal information obtained during the review for any purposes other than for the purpose of conducting the review.

I will keep secure personal information obtained during the review to ensure it is not misused, lost, or improperly accessed, modified or disclosed. After completing the review, I will return to you any documents containing personal information that I obtain from you during the course of the review, except for copies or extracts as required by auditing standards.

Page 2 of 4

Information will not be disclosed by me to other parties except as required or allowed for by law or professional standards, or with your authority. My review files may, however, may be subject to review as part of the quality control review program of The Association of Certified Practicing Accountants.

CPA Australia ("CPAA") which monitors compliance with professional standards by its members. I advise you that by signing this letter you acknowledge that, if requested, my files relating to this review will be made available under either of these review programs. Should this occur I will advise you. The same strict confidentiality requirements apply under the CPAA reviews that apply to myself as your reviewer.

Fees

My fees, which will be billed as work progresses, are based on the time required to complete the engagement, plus direct out-of-pocket expenses. It is policy that my fees be collected within 14 days from the date the invoice was issued, and I trust that this arrangement is acceptable to you.

Please sign and return the attached copy of this letter to indicate that it is in accordance with your understanding of the arrangements for my review.

Yours faithfully,

John Pascoe (FCPA)
Registered Company Audit No. 13479
9/4/18

SIGNED by

CY O'CONNOR ERADE VILLAGE FOUNDATION by its authorised representative

Signature:

Position:

Date:

Page 3 of 4

Auditors Independence Declaration

Under Section 307C of the Corporations Act 2001

To Members of the CY O'Connor Erade Village Foundation

I declare that, to the best of my knowledge and belief, in relation to the audit of the CY O'Connor Erade Village Foundation for the year ended 31 December 2017 there have been:

(a) No contraventions to the auditor independence requirement of the Corporations Act 2001 in relation to the audit; and

(b) No contraventions of any applicable code of professional conduct in relation to the audit.

John Pascoe (FCPA)
Registered Company Audit No. 13479

Dated this NINTH day of APRIL 2018

JOHN D PASCOE, FCPA

Certified Practising Accountant
Registered Tax Agent
Registered Company Auditor

Unit 10/125 Alfred Road
Mount Claremont
Western Australia 6010

ABN 64 724 120 246
Fax: 08 9384 9050
Email:
johnjill@westnet
.com.au Mob:
0406 380 215

5 April 2018

Chairperson
CY O'Connor Erade
Foundation
Level 2/100 Havelock
Street WEST PERTH 6005

Dear Chairperson

INDEPENDENT AUDITOR'S REVIEW REPORT

I have audited the accompanying financial report, being a special purpose financial report of The CY O'Connor Erade Village Foundation (association), which comprises the committee's report, the assets and liabilities statement as at 31 December 2017, the income and expenditure statement for the year ended on, notes comprising a summary of significant accounting policies and other explanatory information and the statement by members of the committee.

Committee's Responsibility for the Financial Report

The committee of The CY O'Connor Erade Village Foundation is responsible for preparation of the financial report, and has determined that the basis of preparation described in Note 1 is appropriate to meet the requirements of the Associations Incorporation Act (1987) and is appropriate to meet the needs of the members. The committee's responsibility also includes such internal control as the committee determines necessary to enable preparation of the financial report that is free from material misstatement, whether due to fraud or error.

Auditor's Responsibility

My responsibility is to express a conclusion on the financial report based on my audit. I conducted my audit in accordance with Auditing Standards. Those standards require that we comply with relevant ethical requirements relating to audit engagements and plan and perform the audit to obtain reasonable assurance whether the financial report is free from material misstatement

An audit involves performing procedures to obtain audit evidence about the amounts and disclosures in the financial report. The procedures selected depend on the auditor's judgement, including the assessment o f the risks of material misstatement of the financial report, whether due to fraud or error. In making those risk assessments, the auditor considers internal control relevant to the association's preparation of the financial report that gives a true and fair view, in order to design audit procedures that are appropriate in the circumstances, but not for the purpose of expressing an opinion on the effectiveness of the association's internal control. An Audit also includes evaluating the appropriateness of accounting policies used and the reasonableness of accounting estimates made by the committee, as well as evaluating the overall presentation of the financial report.

I believe that the audit evidence I have obtained is sufficient and appropriate to provide a basis for the audit opinion.

Qualification

In common with most charitable institutions receiving cash donations, the entity has determined that it is impractical to establish controls over cash donations before they are banked and recorded in the accounting system. As a result my audit was restricted to the amounts recorded in the accounting system.

Opinion

In my opinion, except for the effects on the financial report, if any that the above qualification may have on the financial report of The CY O'Connor Erade Village Foundation, the report presents fairly, in all material respects, the financial position of The CY O'Connor Erade Village Foundation as at 31 December 2017 and its financial performance for the year then ended in accordance with the accounting policies described in Note 1 to the financial statements, and the Associations Incorporation Act (1987).

Basis of Accounting and Restriction on Distribution

Without modifying my opinion, attention is drawn to Note 1 to the financial report, which describes the basis of accounting. The financial report has been prepared to assist The CY O'Connor Erade Village Foundation to meet the requirements of the Associations Incorporation Act (1987). As a result, the financial report may not be suitable for another purpose.

Should you have any queries on the above matter, please do not

hesitate to contact me. Kind regards

John Pascoe (FCPA)
Registered Company Audit No. 13479

Dated this NINTH day of APRIL 2018

Recent Foundation Publications

Genetics of Marbling in Wagyu Revealed by the Melting Temperature of Intramuscular and Subcutaneous Lipids

International Journal of Food Science
Volume 2017, Article ID 3948408, 6 pages
https://doi.org/10.1155/2017/3948408

Sally S. Lloyd,[1,2] *Jose L. Valenzuela,*[1,2,3] *Edward J. Steele,*[1] *and Roger L. Dawkins*[1,2,3]

1 C Y O'Connor ERADE Village Foundation, P.O. Box 5100, Canning Vale South,WA 6155, Australia

2 CY O'Connor Centre for Innovation in Agriculture, Murdoch University, 5 Del Park Road, Box 1, North Dandalup, WA 6207, Australia

3 Melaleuca Stud, 24 Genomics Rise, Piara Waters, WA 6112, Australia

ABSTRACT

Extreme marbling or intramuscular deposition of lipid is associated with Wagyu breeds and is therefore assumed to be largely inherited. However, even within 100% full blood Wagyu prepared under standard conditions, there is unpredictable scatter of the degree of marbling. Here, we evaluate melting temperature (Tm) of intramuscular fat as an alternative to visual scores of marbling. We show that "long fed" Wagyu generally has Tm below body temperature but with a considerable range under standardized conditions. Individual sires have a major impact indicating that the variation is genetic rather than environmental or random error. In order to measure differences of lower marbling breeds and at shorter feeding periods, we have compared Tm in subcutaneous fat samples from over the striploin. Supplementary feeding for 100 to 150 days leads to a rapid decrease in Tm of 50% Red Wagyu (Akaushi): 50% European crosses, when compared to 100% European. This improvement indicates that the genetic effect of Wagyu is useful, predictable, and highly penetrant. Contemporaneous DNA extraction does not affect the measurement of Tm. Thus, provenance can be traced and substitution can be eliminated in a simple and cost-effective manner.

1. Introduction

Marbling (or the accumulation of intramuscular fat) is the holy grail for beef producers, chefs, and their customers, but there is still no agreed definition and therefore no universal standard of measurement [1, 2]. So as to increase commercial returns based on superior taste and health benefits, there have been countless attempts to improve the reproducibility of visual and scanning scores but with limited success [1, 3].

Lipid profiles of highly marbled samples have revealed a high content of oleic acid and therefore a reduction in melting temperature (Tm) [4–6]. A precise and high throughput method for the measurement of Tm exists [7] and is used here to interrogate the complex interplay between the genetic and environmental factors which can be optimized by the producer to the benefit of the health conscious consumer.

Because of the association of Wagyu breeds with high marbling and high oleic acid content, these traits can be assumed to be genetically determined and faithfully inherited [8, 9]. However, in spite of numerous studies [10–19], it has not been possible, hitherto, to identify markers which allow a breeder to quantify superior genetics in individual sires and dams. Some of the explanations for the slow progress include the following:

i) Complexity due to interactions of several metabolic
ii) processes and their regulatory mechanisms [6, 20, 21].
iii) Contribution of many genes with small effects [22].
iv) Uncontrolled environment factors associated with
v) supplementary feeding [23–25].
vi) Difficulty in quantifying marbling reproducibly [2].
vii) Unreliable tracing of meat from paddock to plate.
viii) Perception that fat is dangerous.

Recently it has been demonstrated that that low fat diets have not improved health [26]. In fact, higher oleic acid and therefore low Tm are preferable in terms of lipid profiles [27–29]. This has led to the increasing popularity of the Wagyu brand worldwide. Not surprisingly, mislabeling is now rife resulting in the need to be able to confirm the provenance of retail samples. Here we show that low Tm is heritable and that the same fat sample can be used for the DNA tracing without affecting the measurement of Tm.

2. Materials and Methods

Postmortem samples of meat and fat were taken from carcasses of animals harvested for routine food production. Therefore, ethics approval was not required.

2.1. Dataset 1 Full Blood Wagyu with Identified Sires.

Two cohorts of Wagyu steers (n = 126) were fed for 300 ± 20 days with a proprietary ration within the same commercial feedlot. One-gram samples of meat from the longissimus dorsi were taken from between the 10th and 11th rib. AUSMEAT marbling score (MS) was scored between the 10th and 11th rib, with an average of 7.5 and a range from 2 to 11. Steers for the comparison of sires had their paternity confirmed by DNA testing [30]. Only one progeny of each dam was included so as to focus on the effect of the sire.

2.2. Dataset 2 European and Wagyu Cross Breeds with Varied Feed Time.

Melaleuka Stud, located in the Peel region of Western Australian, 100 km south of Perth, runs a variety of European breeds including Simmental, Gelbvieh, and Angus. This herd was selected to produce high quality beef on pasture, finished with 2 to4months of supplemental feeding. Black and Red Wagyu (full blood or pure bred) have been mated with these European breeds.

Calves stay on milk until 4 months of age when they are weaned and male calves are castrated. After weaning, they continue grazing Kikuyu and Ryegrass pasture until they reach 300 kg. Their feed is then supplemented with 9mm EasyBeef pellets (Milne Feeds, Perth, Australia) ad libitum. The main ingredients of the EasyBeef pellets are lupins, barley, oats, wheat, and triticale. The nutritional composition,

based on dry matter, is crude protein (min) 14.5%, metabolizable energy (est.) 11.0 MJ/kg., crude fiber (max) 20.0%, urea (max) 1.5%, and monensin 26.6 ppm.

The feeders are considered ready for slaughter when they reach a weight of 400 kg and are slaughtered to match demand. Some animals were kept on feed longer to test the effect of increased feeding on Tm and meat quality. The average live weight at slaughter for animals in this study was 461 kg, average age at slaughter was 15.4 months (range 8 to 23), and the average days on feed was 104 days (range 17 to 288). Body numbers from abattoirs were matched to farm records and pedigrees via their RFID tags, where possible identity was confirmed by in-house proprietary DNA testing[30].

Subcutaneous fat overlying the striploin (HAM number 2140) of these cattle was collected after boning and wet aging for 1 to 3 weeks.

2.3. Fat Extraction and Tm Measurement.

Intramuscular fat was extracted from dataset 1 samples by digestion with proteinase K. This method allows for simultaneous extraction of intramuscular fat and DNA from 0.5gram samples of meat if the fat content is above 20%. The samples were incubated at 56∘C, digested in a proteinase K mixture for 4 hours, and centrifuged at 10,000 ×g for 2 minutes to separate the fat from the dissolved DNA and protein solution. Fat was

removed for Tm measurement by pipette. DNA was extracted from the remaining mixture using a standard salting out method.

Intramuscular fat content for many of the carcasses of dataset 2 was too low to allow extraction by the above method. Instead, fat was extracted from 1-gram samples of subcutaneous fat by rendering at 90∘C for at least eight hours.

Samples from 17 sirloin steaks with intramuscular fat higher than 20% were used to determine whether fat separated during a DNA extraction process could be used for *Tm* measurement. Fat was extracted by both digestion and rendering from the same samples and the *Tm* measurements compared.

Tm of all fat samples was determined in triplicate according to the thermocycler method [7], which is closely correlated to slip points, although the values are higher by 2∘C for animal fat with a *Tm* of 40∘C.

3. Results

3.1. Tm Is Affected by Sire.

Samples were taken from long fed Wagyu steers differing only by sire and dam (dataset 1). The steers were fed, harvested, and tested in two cohorts two months apart. The cohorts did not differ significantly in feeding, genetics, or initial *Tm* (as shown in

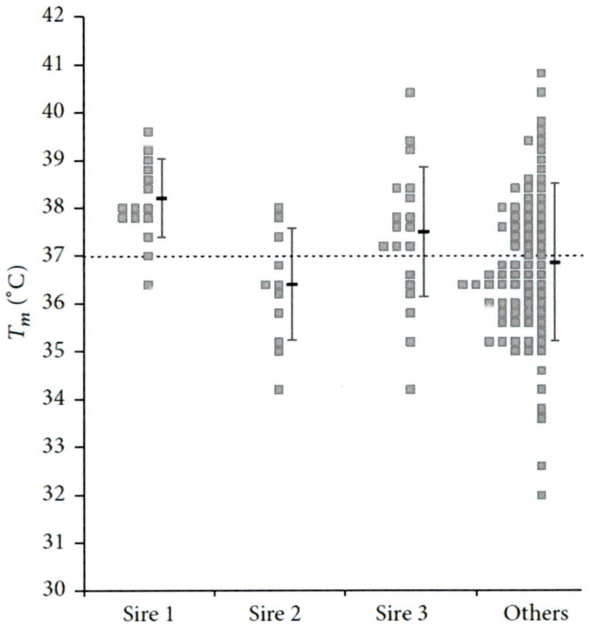

Figure 1: ⍰⍰ distributions of Wagyu carcasses differ by sire.The melting temperature of intramuscular fat samples taken from between the 10th and 11th ribof 126 carcasses of full blood Wagyu steers. All animalswere fed the same ration for 300±20 days. Individual ⍰⍰ measurements of carcasses are grouped by sire (mean and standard deviation). Animals with either an uncertain sire or a sire with less than 10 progeny aregrouped under "other" sires. Progeny of Sire 3 shows considerable scatter, whereas 8/11 of those of Sire 2 are below 37 degrees compared with 1/15 in the case of Sire 1.The difference between Sire 1 and Sire 2 is statistically significant with a chi-square statistic of 12.2 and thus a ⍰ value < 0.01.

Supplemental Table 1 in Supplementary Material available online at https://doi.org/10.1155 /2017/3948408) and have therefore been combined for further analysis. *Tm* and marble score were analyzed by sire for the three sires with more than ten progenies. As shown in Figure 1, *Tm* of the progeny of Sire 2 fell consistently, whereas Sire 1 had little impact. In fact, 14 progenies of Sire 1 were above 37∘C, compared to only 3 of Sire 2. The cross-product ratio is 104/6 or 17, as shown in Figure 1. This difference is highly significant (p value < 0.01 by $\chi 2$). It is noteworthy that there is more scatter with Sire 3 and all
remaining sires. By contrast with *Tm*, visual scores of marbling gave greater scatter, did not demonstrate a sire effect, and must be misleading in their present form.

3.2. In Wagyu, Tm Falls with Days on Feed and Proportion of Wagyu.

Notwithstanding the genetic effects, there is also a major

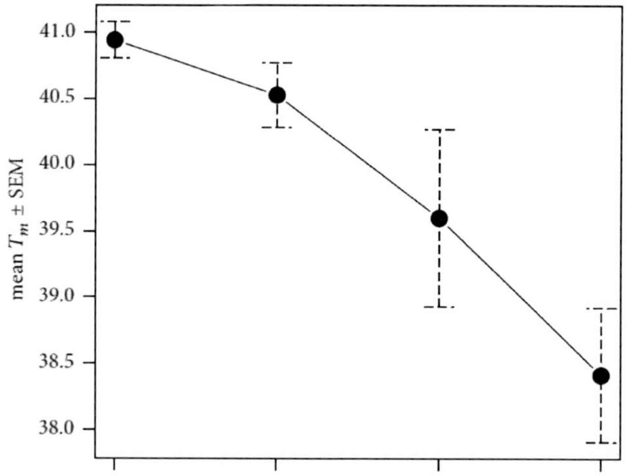

Breed	EU100	WY25	WY50	WY75+
N	176	29	11	15
DOF Mean ± SD	84 ± 41	103 ± 52	167 ± 103	225 ± 79

Figure 2: □□ decreases with feeding and increasing proportion of Wagyu ancestry. □□ of subcutaneous fat samples over the loin of a mix of breeds and crossbreeds including Simmental, Gelbvieh, Angus, Dexter, andWagyu. 176 samples (EU100) came from 100% European breeds fed for an average of 81 days. WY25, WY50, and WY75+ samples had 25%, 50%, and 75–100% Wagyu ancestry, respectively.There were 29 samples ofWY25, 14 samples ofWY50, and 11 samples of WY75+ with average days on feed of 103, 167, and 225, respectively.

environmental effect on *Tm* and marbling. *Tm* results of dataset 2, grouped by proportion of black Wagyu, are shown in Figure 2. *Tm* falls with increase in Wagyu and days on feed. Separating these two variables is not yet possible but, in the meanwhile, the results suggest that increasing the content of Wagyu genes allows the benefit of long feeding. The European cattle included in this study do not show the same benefit as the Wagyu.
Importantly, the benefits are seen with only 25% Wagyu, again emphasizing the high penetrance of the Wagyu genetics.

3.3. Quantitative Effect of Feeding.
So as to address the complex interaction between genetics and environment, we compared two breed groups from dataset 2: a control group of purely European cattle (EU100) and the F1 Red Wagyu, also known as Akaushi and recorded as AK50. The dams have a similar breed composition and history to the EU100 control group. So as to avoid the complexity of sampling intramuscular fat before it is visible, we have relied on *Tm* measurements of overlying

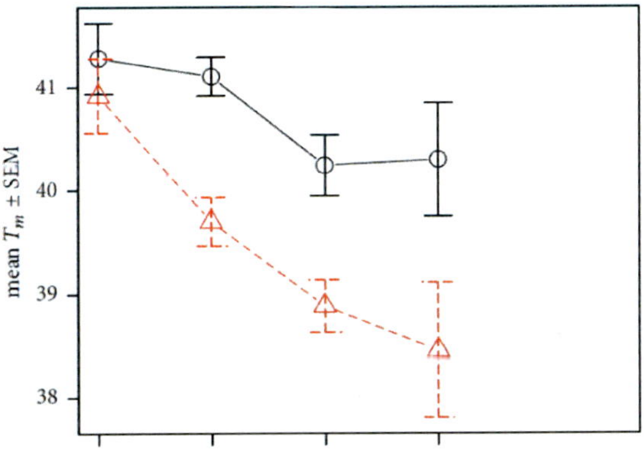

Days on feed	1 to 50	51 to 100	101 to 150	Over 150
Number of EU100	26	84	34	9
Number of AK50	5	33	31	7

Breed
EU100
AK50

Figure 3: RedWagyu sired carcasses have lower ⍰⍰ for equivalent DOF. ⍰⍰ was measured for subcutaneous fat samples taken from the loins of 229 carcasses.The cattle were backgrounded on pasture and then fed on pellets until they reached a satisfactory weight and fatness.The results are grouped by days on feed and by breed of sire (European or Akaushi).The dams of all carcasses were European breeds. Breed and days on feed were both statistically significant influences on ⍰⍰, with ⍰ < 0.01 calculated by multiway ANOVA. The difference between the two groups was significant after only 51–100 days on feed.

subcutaneous fat. The effect of feeding is clear as shown in Figure 3. *Tm* falls progressively even with only a 50% infusion of Akaushi.

3.4.DNA Extraction Does Not Invalidate Measurement of Tm.
In Figure 4 we show that extracting DNA with the proteinase K does not affect the measurement of *Tm* on the same extract. Oxidation of the polyunsaturated fatty acids in the sample that may have occurred during rendering at 90∘C did not have a measurable effect on the melting point, as expected [4, 31].

4. Discussion

The intention of these studies is to resolve, in part, the manifest
confusion facing producers and consumers of healthy beef.
It is clear that Wagyu beef is superior, as reflected by the commercial returns for highly marbled beef, but increasingly

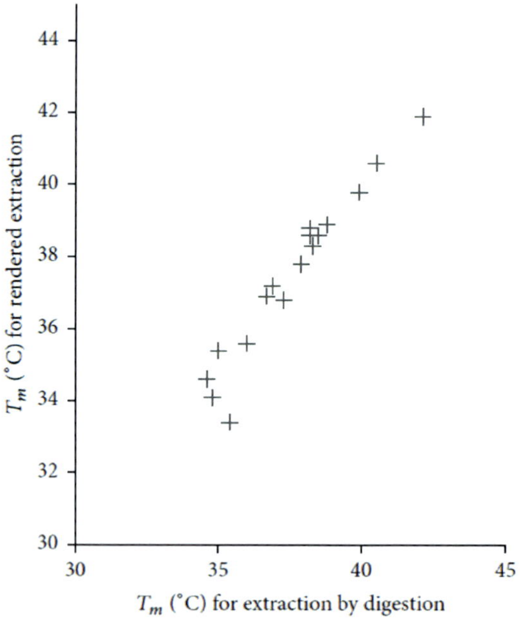

Figure 4: Simultaneous extraction of fat and DNA does not change ▯▯. There is excellent correlation between ▯▯ measurements of fat harvested during DNA and extracted by rendering (Pearson's ▯ = 0.97). There was no measurable bias (mean difference 0.13, SEM = 0.14). Either extraction method can be used for direct comparison without adjustment.

the brand is amenable to misuse.
A major issue is the lack of a reproducible measurement of the degree of marbling. Multiple and incompatible systems of scoring may have been retained perhaps to the advantage of some sectors. The measurement of Tm is possible at successive stages of the production line so that quality can be confirmed. At the same time, DNA can be extracted so that provenance can be confirmed.
The difficulty faced by the breeder is even more important. Nonreproducible measurement obfuscates attempt to identify breeding values and therefore confound selection of superior sires. This issue becomes particularly important in an attempt to upgrade first crosses. The present results show that even WY25 can have reduced Tm but the scatter is substantial leading to lack of consistency. Future studies may identify those sires which are well suited to crossbreeding.
So as to reduce the number of variables we sampled AK50 at differing days on feed. All had European dams. The initial results are promising in that there was a progressive decline in Tm. Further work may define the preferred type and length of supplementary feeding. Importantly, there is also the potential to examine the controversies surrounding the use of grass versus grain. Whilst there is growing consumer demand for less intensive feeding and especially for "grassfed," there is also the perception that corn and perhaps other grains are necessary for extreme marbling. Given reproducible measurements, it should be possible to define acceptable compromises between supplementation, on the one hand, and tastiness and healthiness, on the other hand.
A major finding of this study is the difference in Tm between the progeny of two full blood Wagyu sires. Sire 1 and Sire 2 share a paternal and a maternal grand sire and were imported from the same prefecture in Japan. Pedigree analysis alone would not predict large differences in lipid composition. It is noteworthy however that Sire 1 and Sire 2 are quite different in their C19 haplotypes, as described elsewhere [32]. A major issue remains unresolved. The degree of marbling and the lipid profile differ depending upon the site of sampling; as an approximation the intramuscular accumulation of lipid progress from the brisket backwards with the more caudal fat deposits having somewhat lower proportions of oleic acid and higher Tm [33]. Therefore, comparable samples need to be

from a fixed location. Even within the same muscle group there is variation depending upon sampling [34]. We recommend further experience using subcutaneous fat so that its utility can be extended. Ultimately, it should be possible to take in vivo samples so as to monitor changes with time, genetics, and feed.

Conflicts of Interest

Collectively, the authors associated with the CY O'Connor ERADE Village Foundation have an interest in the work described in this manuscript as it forms part of the foundation's
intellectual property.

Acknowledgments

The authors are grateful to the collaboration of breeders who provided samples and to Dom Bayard, Scott de Bruin, Peter Gilmour, Keith Hammond, Bruce Cheung, Alan Peggs, Bob Reed, Graham Truscott, Carel Tesling, J. R. Dawkins, and Lindsay Baker for advice and suggestions. This is publication 1504 of the CY O'Connor ERADE Village Foundation supported by funding from Pardoo Pastoral and Melaleuka Stud.

References

[1] W. Cheng, J. H. Cheng, D.W. Sun, and H. Pu, "Marbling Analysis for Evaluating Meat Quality: Methods and Techniques," Comprehensive Reviews in Food Science and Food Safety, vol. 14, no. 5, pp. 523–535, 2015.

[2] D. D. Johnson, J. W. Savell, D. M. Stiffler, and H. R. Cross, "Postmortem environmental factors affecting beef carcass lean maturity and marbling evaluations," Journal of Food Quality, vol. 8, pp. 253–264, 1986.

[3] K. Kuchida, S. Kono, K. Konishi, L. D. Van Vleck, M. Suzuki, and S. Miyoshi, "Prediction of crude fat content of longissimus muscle of beef using the ratio of fat area calculated from computer image analysis: Comparison of regression equations for prediction using different input devices at different stations," Journal of Animal Science, vol. 78, no. 4, pp. 799–803, 2000.

[4] K. Y. Chung, D. K. Lunt, C. B. Choi et al., "Lipid characteristics of subcutaneous adipose tissue and M. longissimus thoracis of Angus and Wagyu steers fed to US and Japanese endpoints," Meat Science, vol. 73, no. 3, pp. 432–441, 2006.

[5] S. De Smet, K. Raes, and D. Demeyer, "Meat fatty acid composition as affected by fatness and genetic factors: a review," Animal Research, vol. 53, no. 2, pp. 81–98, 2004.

[6] S. B. Smith, C. A. Gill, D. K. Lunt, and M. A. Brooks, "Regulation of fat and fatty acid composition in beef cattle," Asian- Australasian Journal of Animal Sciences, vol. 22, no. 9, pp. 1225– 1233, 2009.

[7] S. S. Lloyd, S. T. Dawkins, and R. L.Dawkins, "Anovel method ofmeasuring the melting point of animal fats," Journal ofAnimal Science, vol. 92, no. 10, pp. 4775–4778, 2014.
[8] M. Zembayashi, K. Nishimura, D. K. Lunt, and S. B. Smith, "Effect of breed type and sex on the fatty acid composition of subcutaneous and intramuscular lipids of finishing steers and heifers.," Journal of Animal Science, vol. 73, no. 11, pp. 3325–3332, 1995.
[9] A. E. O. Malau-Aduli, M. A. Edriss, B. D. Siebert, C. D. K. Bottema, andW. S. Pitchford, "Breed differences and genetic parameters for melting point, marbling score and fatty acid composition of lot-fed cattle," Journal of Animal Physiology and Animal Nutrition, vol. 83, no. 2, pp. 95–105, 2000.
[10] L. Barto˘n, D. Bure˘s, T. Kott, and D. ˘Reh´ak, "Associations of polymorphisms in bovine DGAT1, FABP4, FASN, and PPARGC1A genes with intramuscular fat content and the fatty acid composition of muscle and subcutaneous fat in Fleckvieh bulls," Meat Science, vol. 114, pp. 18–23, 2016.
[11] H. S.Cheong,D.Yoon, L. H.Kimet al., "Titin-cap (TCAP) polymorphisms associated with marbling score of beef," Meat Science, vol. 77, no. 2, pp. 257–263, 2007.
[12] C. Han,M. Vinsky, N. Aldai, M. E. R. Dugan, T. A. McAllister, and C. Li, "Association analyses of DNA polymorphisms in bovine SREBP-1, LXRα, FADS1 genes with fatty acid composition in Canadian commercial crossbred beef steers," Meat Science, vol. 93, no. 3, pp. 429–436, 2013.
[13] J. Papaleo Mazzucco, D. E. Goszczynski, M. V. Ripoli et al., "Growth, carcass and meat quality traits in beef from Angus, Hereford and cross-breed grazing steers, and their association with SNPs in genes related to fat deposition metabolism," Meat Science, vol. 114, pp. 121–129, 2016.
[14] L. Xu, L. P. Zhang, Z. R. Yuan et al., "Polymorphismof SREBP1 is associated with beef fatty acid composition in Simmental bulls," Genetics and Molecular Research, vol. 12, no. 4, pp. 5802–5809, 2013.
[15] S. Zhang, T. J. Knight, J. M. Reecy, and D. C. Beitz, "DNA polymorphisms in bovine fatty acid synthase are associated with beef fatty acid composition," Animal Genetics, vol. 39, no. 1, pp. 62–70, 2008.
[16] M. Shibata, K. Matsumoto, K. Aikawa, T. Muramoto, S. Fujimura, and M. Kadowaki, "Gene expression of myostatin during development and regeneration of skeletal muscle in Japanese Black Cattle," Journal of Animal Science, vol. 84, no. 11, pp. 2983–2989, 2006.
[17] M. Saatchi, D. J. Garrick, R. G. Tait et al., "Genome-wide association and prediction of direct genomic breeding values for composition of fatty acids in Angus beef cattlea," BMC Genomics, vol. 14, no. 1, article no. 730, 2013.
[18] T.Matsuhashi, S.Maruyama, Y.Uemoto et al., "Effects of bovine fatty acid synthase, stearoyl-coenzyme A desaturase, sterol regulatory element-binding protein 1, and growth hormone gene polymorphisms on fatty acid composition and carcass traits in Japanese Black cattle," Journal of Animal Science, vol. 89, no. 1, pp. 12–22, 2011.
[19] K. Hayakawa, T. Sakamoto, A. Ishii et al., "The g.841G>C SNP of FASN gene is associated with fatty acid composition in beef cattle," Journal of Animal Science, pp. 737–746, 2015.

[20] P. McGilchrist, D. W. Pethick, S. P. F. Bonny, P. L. Greenwood, and G. E. Gardner, "Whole body insulin responsiveness is higher in beef steers selected for increased muscling," Animal, vol. 5, no. 10, pp. 1579–1586, 2011.
[21] P. McGilchrist, D. W. Pethick, S. P. F. Bonny, P. L. Greenwood, and G. E. Gardner, "Beef cattle selected for increasedmuscularity have a reducedmuscle response and increased adipose tissue response to adrenaline," Animal, vol. 5, no. 6, pp. 875–884, 2011.
[22] W. G.Hill, "Applications of population genetics to animal breeding, fromwright, fisher and lush to genomic prediction," Genetics, vol. 196, no. 1, pp. 1–16, 2014.
[23] P. R. Myer, T. P. L. Smith, J. E. Wells, L. A. Kuehn, and H. C. Freetly, "Rumen microbiome from steers differing in feed efficiency," PLoS ONE, vol. 10, no. 6, Article IDe0129174, 2015.
[24] Z.Durmic, P. J. Moate, R. Eckard, D. K. Revell, R.Williams, and P. E. Vercoe, "In vitro screening of selected feed additives, plant essential oils and plant extracts for rumenmethane mitigation," Journal of the Science of Food and Agriculture, vol. 94, no. 6, pp. 1191–1196, 2014.
[25] Z. Durmic, C. S. McSweeney, G. W. Kemp, P.Hutton, R. J. Wallace, andP. E. Vercoe, "Australianplantswithpotential to inhibit bacteria and processes involved in ruminal biohydrogenation of fatty acids," Animal Feed Science and Technology, vol. 145, no. 1- 4, pp. 271–284, 2008.
[26] N. Teicholz, A Big Fat Surprise, Simon and Schuster,New York, NY, USA, 2014.
[27] T. H. Adams, R. L. Walzem, D. R. Smith, S. Tseng, and S. B. Smith, "Hamburger high in total, saturated and trans-fatty acids decreasesHDL cholesterol and LDL particle diameter, and increases TAG, in mildly hypercholesterolaemic men," British Journal of Nutrition, vol. 103, no. 1, pp. 91–98, 2010.
[28] L. A.Gilmore, R. L.Walzem, S. F.Crouse et al., "Consumption of high-oleic acid ground beef increases HDL-cholesterol concentration but both high- and low-oleic acid ground beef decrease HDL particle diameter in normocholesterolemic men," Journal of Nutrition, vol. 141, no. 6, pp. 1188–1194, 2011.
[29] R. P. Mensink, P. L. Zock, A. D. Kester, andM. B. Katan, "Effects of dietary fatty acids and carbohydrates on the ratio of serum total to HDL cholesterol and on serum lipids and apolipoproteins: a meta-analysis of 60 controlled trials," American Journal of Clinical Nutrition, vol. 77, no. 5, pp. 1146–1155, 2003.
[30] J. F.Williamson, E. J. Steele, S. Lester et al., "Genomic evolution in domestic cattle: Ancestral haplotypes and healthy beef," Genomics, vol. 97, no. 5, pp. 304–312, 2011.
[31] J. D. Wood, R. I. Richardson, G. R. Nute et al., "Effects of fatty acids on meat quality: a review," Meat Science, vol. 66, no. 1, pp. 21–32, 2004.
[32] S. S. Lloyd, E. J. Steele, J. L. Valenzuela, and R. L. Dawkins, "Haplotypes for type, degree, and rate of marbling in cattle are syntenic with human muscular dystrophy," International Journal of Genomics, vol. 2017, 14 pages, 2017.
[33] S. B. Smith and B. J. Johnson, Marbling: Management of cattle to maximize the deposition of intramuscular adipose tissue, National cattlemens beef association, Centennial, 2014.

[34] Y. Nakahashi, S.Maruyama, S. Seki, S. Hidaka, and K. Kuchida, "Relationships between monounsaturated fatty acids of marbling flecks and image analysis traits in longissimus muscle for Japanese Black steers," Journal of Animal Science, vol. 86, no. 12, pp. 3551–3556, 2008.

Haplotypes for Type, Degree and Rate of Marbling in Cattle are Syntenic with Human Muscular Dystrophy.

Published 2017, International Journal of Genomics, Article ID 6532837

Sally S Lloyd[1,2,3], *Edward J Steele*[1], *Jose L Valenzuela*[1,2] *and Roger L Dawkins*[1,2,3]*

[1]CY O'Connor ERADE Village Foundation, PO Box 5100 Canning Vale South, Western Australia, Australia 6155
[2]Melaleuka Stud, 24 Genomics Rise, Piara Waters, Western Australia, Australia 6112
[3]Centre for Innovation in Agriculture, Murdoch University, Murdoch, Western Australia, Australia 6150
*Corresponding Author

ABSTRACT

Traditional analyses of a QTL on Bota 19 implicate a surfeit of candidates, but each is of marginal significance in explaining the deposition of healthy, low melting temperature fat within marbled muscle of Wagyu cattle.

As an alternative approach, we have used genomic, multigenerational segregation to identify 14 conserved, ancestral 20Mb haplotypes. These determine the degree and rate of marbling in Wagyu and other breeds of cattle.

The melting temperature of intramuscular fat is highly heritable and traceable by haplotyping. Fortunately, for the production of healthy beef, some of these haplotypes are sufficiently penetrant to be expressed in heterozygous crossbreds, thereby allowing selection of sires which will improve the healthiness of beef produced under even harsh climatic conditions.

The region of Bota 19 is syntenic to a region of Hosa 17 known to be important in muscle metabolism and in determining susceptibility to a form of human muscular dystrophy.

INTRODUCTION

Conserved Ancestral Haplotypes have been highly informative in revealing the functional significance of polymorphic sequences especially when extensive enough to encode

regulatory regions as well as structural elements. [1–3]
In Homo sapiens (Hosa), there are now many examples of conserved haplotypes regulating the degree of expression of a trait or disease such as an enzyme deficiency, immune competence, drug reactions and disease severity. The best known examples are the extended haplotypes of the Major Histocompatibility Complex[1,2,4–7] but the principle applies throughout the genome,[8] with the important caveat that the haplotypes are identified and tagged correctly.[9,10] Many of these haplotypes were discovered through the finding of genetic associations with quantitative traits, such as diseases. It became obvious that there are tens or even hundreds of alternative haplotypes encoding functionally important regions of the genome and that these interact with each other positively or negatively. A potent example is IgA deficiency[2,6,11–13] which is associated with the 8.1 haplotype *inter alia.* The precise mechanisms underlying this regulatory defect are not clear from analysis of SNPs and coding sequences.[14]
For the breeding of livestock, it is traditional [15,16] to follow the precepts of the infinitesimal model which assumes there are independent genes separated by free recombination.[17] However it is quite clear that this assumption is not correct.[3,17] The genomic architecture of cattle,[18–21] sheep,[22,23] goats,[24] dogs, [25,26] mice, [27] and pigs[28,29] is remarkably similar to that present in Hosa, where there are kilobase and even megabase blocks of polymorphism at which there are retroviral and other indels, segmental duplications and differences in copy number in addition to nucleotide substitutions.[1,2,30,31]
In cattle, there are many traits of proven importance to the production of healthy food. There have been numerous attempts to find useful genetic markers if only for selection of superior breeding pairs for commercial gain. Results have been disappointing for several reasons generally reflecting an over-simplified understanding of the genomic structure. Thus, conserved ancestral haplotypes can be confounding if not identified. For example, desirable traits such as increased milk production can be associated with disadvantages such as infertility.[3] In other instances, the genetic marker may appear useful in one breed but not another, as illustrated by polling.[3]

Here we address these disappointments by identifying megabase haplotypes of critical interest to healthy food and public health[32,33] and potential relevance to the metabolic changes underlying limb girdle muscular dystrophy.
True or fine marbling describes the deposition of lipid between and within muscle fibres as occurs after supplementary feeding for a year or more. The genesis is very complex, including differentiation of satellite or progenitor cells, and is obviously tightly regulated,[34] but the ultimate effect is to improve taste and juiciness thereby increasing the value of beef several fold. More importantly, marbling increases the content of the healthy, monounsaturated fatty acid (MUFA) and is therefore "cholesterol lowering" and statin-sparing.[35,36] These features are characteristic of Japanese cattle, known as Wagyu, Black and Red, but may be found to lesser degrees in other breeds and crossbreeds. It is important to distinguish true or fine marbling from the deposition of subcutaneous and interfascicular fat as is characteristic of European breeds.
For more than 20 years, initially in Japan, there have been attempts to find predictors of:

- How much a given animal will marble,
- Which matings are preferable, and
- Whether the very costly feeding can be reduced?

At face value, the results are contradictory but also tantalising since the inconsistencies may be due to the complexity of the marbling pathway and the sheer number of genes involved.
A simple polymorphism of the SCD (delta-9 desaturase on Bota 26) appears to affect the amount of marbling presumably by encouraging desaturation and therefore the production of MUFA and particularly oleic acid. Polymorphisms of Growth Hormone (GH) and Fatty Acid Synthase (FASN) amongst many others, may also have an effect. The evidence for some of these individual genes is reviewed and presented in Table 1. [37–54] From these 14 studies the only fair conclusion is that, although the genomic region controls fat deposition, multiple genes and therefore haplotypes must be involved.
Our interest increased when it became apparent that a regulator of SCD, SREBF1, maps to the Bota 19 chromosome together with GH and FASN. Taken with the pleiotropic regulatory role of SREBF1, in humans at least, [55] and with the evidence for the influence of Bota 19 on fatty acid

composition in Japanese Black cattle,[48,49] we asked whether extensive, multi-megabase haplotypes could be identified. Previous investigations [37–54] have suggested that some intervening and adjacent genes could be relevant. Such apparent clustering of plausible candidates is often illusory, but in this case, we were encouraged by the fact that Japanese breeders are sufficiently convinced to be prepared to pay handsomely for SCD and GH typing even though it seems clear that these genes are unlikely to be involved directly.

Accordingly, we have been defining conserved ancestral haplotypes within the region. The many conserved megabase haplotypes have very different frequencies when breeds are compared.[56] The need for a simple summary of breed differences led to development of the W plots which separate haplotypes common to all cattle from those which are found in, and potentially defining for, one breed but not the other.[57,58]Of course, since Wagyu cattle marble, it follows that all Wagyu specific haplotypes must be associated with marbling irrespective of their function; all too often, such passive associations have been misinterpreted as causal. Common haplotypes may be implicated unless non-marbling breeds are compared to determine which are specific for marbling breeds. The challenge is to assess the Wagyu haplotypes in different backgrounds such as can be obtained by crossing Wagyu with other breeds which are relatively resistant to marbling.

As a strategy, we asked whether Wagyu specific haplotypes, once defined, are penetrant when heterozygous in F1 crossbreds. If so, it would be fair to conclude that these haplotypes have direct effects on the marbling process. We also asked whether non-Wagyu haplotypes affect the *rate* of marbling alone or in combination. Therefore, we started the investigation by determining whether fine marbling of progeny is a function of parentage.

In order to undertake such studies, it is critical to have a reliable measurement of marbling. In spite of many attempts, including use of photographic and ultrasound images, there is still no agreed international benchmark, largely because the deposition of the preferred fat is very fine and barely visible. The most objective approach is the cumbersome slip test for the measurement of melting temperature (T_m) of the lipid fraction and effectively the predominance of oleic acid.[34,59]In Wagyu, T_ms below body temperature (37°C) correlate with fine marbling thereby explaining the cholesterol lowering and statin sparing effects.[34]

We have introduced a more convenient and highly reproducible variation using the same thermocycler as used for the Polymerase Chain Reaction.[60]

With this method, elsewhere we will show that low T_m is highly heritable as expected given its extreme expression in only the Wagyu breed. Furthermore, we show that the effect is determined by multiple, conserved, megabase haplotypes. These can be used to predict marbling in crossbreds. There is evidence for *cis* interactions within, and *trans* interactions between, haplotypes. We also describe a strategy for improving the quality and healthiness of beef by judicious crossing.

The step-wise approach used here can be applied to other challenges in livestock genetics especially where regulatory ancestral haplotypes are suspected. Systematically, we address:

- Synteny as a guide to functions and interactions already defined in Hosa.
- Breed effects as an initial screen for heritability.
- Heritability as the only variable
- Genomic markers of inheritance
- Haplotypes in crossbreds
- Mechanisms of haplotype effects

The conclusions of all these complementary studies lead to a model of the genetic control of fatty acid composition.

RESULTS

Synteny as a Guide

In Figure 1 we show the regions of Hosa chr17 which correspond to SREBF1 to FASN on Bota chr 19. Note also the regulatory effects of SREBF1 on remote sites many of which map closely with locations implicated in limb girdle muscular dystrophy.

In the dot plot of GH to FASN it is apparent that there are two separate components in Hosa; the blue and green sections are distinct but note how they remain contiguous even though the green has been inverted. Similar phenomena are present elsewhere in the synteny plot. Together these suggest that there are multiple interacting haplotypes from SREBF1 to

FASN.

Breed Effects and Heritability

Most Wagyu have T_m of intramuscular fat below human body temperature of 37°C and distinctly lower than fat from Simmentals which is mostly subcutaneous and generally above 40°C [60]. The length of feeding was much greater for Wagyu due to the fact that the Simmentals grow rapidly and fatten quickly through deposition of largely subcutaneous fat. Wagyu are much slower to both grow and fatten as they deposit intramuscular rather than subcutaneous fat.

We compared Wagyu cattle with various European breeds and crossbreeds which were fed the same ration under the same environmental conditions, but with days on feed varied to achieve the desired finish. The results showed that the Tm of subcutaneous fat was lower in animals with higher proportions of wagyu ancestry. (data not shown here). Differences were noticeable in animals with only 25% Wagyu ancestry indicating that the breed effect can be highly penetrant.

Wagyu steers were fed together for 300 days and assessed identically. The only significant variable was parentage which was confirmed by DNA haplotyping. All sires are considered to be elite in terms of their breeding, reputation and Estimated Breeding Value (EBV) when available. The progeny groups differ significantly, with mean T_m for the progeny of two sires differing by nearly 2 degrees. Importantly, this effect was not seen with the visual marbling score. There is an unequivocal genetic effect detectable within one generation. Thus, in spite of the undoubted complexity of the inheritance, sires can be ranked according to heritability of low T_m.

Thus, breed differences, individual sires and presumably identifiable genetic factors, determine the type, rate and location of lipid deposition. However, it is also clear that there is major effect of environment in that T_m falls with increasing DOF irrespective of breed and this fact compounded by imprecision may have contributed to past confusion.
In the analysis of genetic differences presented here we define alleles and haplotypes common in wagyu but rare in other breeds that may explain some of the differences in the type, rate and location of lipid deposition.

Genomic Markers of Inheritance

The genomic structure of the relevant region of Bota 19 contains the previously implicated SREBF1 and GH, as shown in Figures 1 and 2. Note the extensive duplication as found in other genomic regions of polymorphism including differences in copy number. The degree of polymorphism (at the insensitive gel level) ranges from at least 7 alleles at the most polymorphic locus (MPRIP) and to only 2 at the least (TCAP). In the SREBF1 to GH (S-G) segment there are 3 x 5 x 7 x 2 x 3 = 630 possible haplotypes on each paternal or maternal chromosome. Therefore, there should be some thousands of genotypes if the alleles at each locus are segregating randomly due to free recombination as specified in the infinitesimal model of population genetics.

Here we report the actual frequencies in Wagyu and in some of the breeds with which they have been crossed. Only 14 haplotypes occur commonly, say greater than 5%, in the breeds studied here. Importantly, as shown in Figure 3 and Figure 4, these are the conserved ancestral haplotypes. Four of the fourteen are present in the three generation family which also shows the segregation of the *a* haplotype in three genotypes. None of the haplotypes could be identified through linkage disequilibrium; they must be observed empirically. They are NOT recent recombinants or mutants. They are NOT those expected from the allele frequencies and random assortment. Random segregation and free recombination can be excluded at least in this 20 megabase region.

As shown in Figure 2, haplotypes are designated by the alleles at MPRIP, TCAP, SREBF1 and NT5M in that order so as emphasize the conservation over the 5 megabases between MPRIP and TCAP (M-T segment). Note in Figure 1 that MPRIP and TCAP are adjacent in Bota but not Hosa.

The 60.10.S.10 is the most common Wagyu-specific haplotype. Other haplotypes are found in all breeds (e.g. 30.20.L.20 and 40.20.L.20) and yet others are characteristic of a breed such as Simmental (e.g. 30.10.L.10). These breed differences are shown as a W plot in Figure 4.

It can be seen that the conserved ancestral haplotypes extend from SREBF1 to FASN. The breed differences are especially striking at GH and FASN. Note that Wagyu specific haplotypes have L at FASN whereas Simmental specific haplotypes have S (Figure 4a), This remarkable difference might suggest that FASN is critical, but similar breed specificity is apparent at GH. Further, an association with 60.10.S.10.B.L or 30.20.S.20.C.L in Wagyu could be misinterpreted as implicating the shared alleles SREBF1 S or FASN L which are megabases apart. Note also that the remarkable but unpredictable associations between alleles at SREBF1, GH and FASN have the potential to explain why there has been 20 years of confusion and argument as to which particular gene is important. As also shown in Figure 4a the five haplotypes in the family are also present in the W plot. Three are essentially Wagyu specific whereas two are common to cattle generally implying conservation over at least thousands of generations.

By comparing the haplotypes in the Red and Black Wagyu it can be seen that the 60.10 segment at M-T is shared but the SREBF1 to NTM5 (S-N) segments differ (see Figure 2). Both types of Wagyu are known for their fine marbling suggesting that M-T crucial.

Haplotypes in crossbreds

A key question is which Wagyu haplotypes can have an effect in crossbreds when the genetic background is foreign. Samples were taken from exhibits submitted to a steak competition intended to compare production systems rather than genetics. The results of T_m measurements are shown in Figure 5. The fullbloods are below 36°C in 7/9 as expected. Although the crossbreds, taken as a group, have higher T_m, remarkably, 4/16 are below 36°C. Of the 11/16 crossbreds with T_m m below 38°C, 9/11 have one or the other of two *Wagyu specific* haplotypes. Thus, these two haplotypes (60.10.S.10 and 30.20.S.20) are associated with, if not directly responsible for, the dramatic fall in T_m obtained by crossing a high T_m breed with a Black Wagyu which transmits one of these haplotypes. Note that these two haplotypes differ in the M-T segment but share S at SREBF1.

So as to examine the effect of haplotypes in another setting, we compared Marbling Scores in cross breds differing by whether they inherited haplotypes classified as specific for either wagyu or bos indicus. As shown in Table 3, the former group had greater marbling.

Mapping mechanisms to haplotypes

It is unrealistic to expect to map single functions to ancestral haplotypes as if these were just a string of bi-allelic coding genes. The sequence conservation is so extensive, so complex and, as yet, so poorly understood! However, it is reasonable to expect that the differences will be quantitative and that penetrance will be dependent on multiple variables. At minimum, there will be multiple *cis* and *trans* interactions between the various polymorphisms. It follows that we expect to find associations at multiple markers. The results given above appear to implicate sequences around S and within the M-T segment of Wagyu haplotypes irrespective of effects marked by GH and FASN (see Figure 2).

In order to evaluate such conclusions and so as to assess other markers and haplotypes, we have taken advantage of the availability of two very different data sets:
Mayura – Fixed environment including 300 DOF, 100% black Wagyu, permitting examination of genetic differences within black Wagyu.
Melaleuka – Fixed environment but variable DOF and breed, permitting examination of all haplotypes, Wagyu haplotypes within crossbreds and effects on the *rate* of marbling
Table 2 gives some of the results of the Mayura set. As already shown, see Figure 4, this is the set which revealed the heritability of T_m confirming its value in dissecting complex genetics. For convenience, we show a cut-off of 37°C, giving approximately 50% in the above and below groups. By comparing alleles at four of the loci shown in Figure 2, it is clear that the TCAP 20 allele is associated with lower T_m. The MPRIP 60 is associated with higher T_m. Although SREBF1 S is a marker for low T_m in some earlier studies and patents, here we find the opposite. At the NT5M locus, the 22 allele is associated with low T_m.

The inconsistencies between past and present results and between locus *versus* haplotype analysis can be illustrated as follows. The prototypic Wagyu ancestral sequence, 60.10.S10, can be recognized by the 60.10.S.10 combination, but these alleles, taken individually, are ***not*** haplospecific. As shown in Figure 2, each is found on more than one haplotype.

When the alleles are examined without regard to whether they are carried by the ancestral haplotype, T_m would be a higher, higher, higher and higher at MPRIP, TCAP, SREB-P and NT5M respectively (see Table 2). However, as shown in Figure 5, the 60.10.S.10 ancestral haplotype actually lowers the T_m of crossbreds. Thus, there may be multiple *cis* and *trans* interactions contributing to the effect of a particular haplotype.

As a further approach to address the complexity, we asked whether there is any influence of *trans* interaction or homozygosity. Since it would be necessary to study many hundreds of thousands of individuals to obtain sufficient homozygotes of even the most common haplotypes, we chose to examine the least polymorphic loci such as TCAP with only two alleles:10 and 20. In the Mayura long-fed Wagyu data set, all 8 with T_m below 36°C are 20,20 homozygotes (see Figure 6). Using 37°C as a cut-off, 60% of 20,20 are lower compared with only 33% of the 10,10 homozygotes.
The effect of TCAP homozygosity is clear in a genetically very diverse group fed for 450 days. Only subcutaneous fat from over the rump was available. Although not comparable to other samples reported above, TCAP 10,10 homozygotes have higher Tm than 20,20 homozygotes (Table 4).
So as to address the issue in a very different data set, we analised the Melaleuka Euro and Crossbred cattle and found similar results. As shown in Figure 7, TCAP 10,10 and 20,20 homozygotes diverge after 50-100 DOF. After 100 DOF, 9 of 12 with TCAP 10,10 remain above 39°C compared with 3 of 12 with TCAP 20,20. ($p < 0.05$). The 20,20 homozygotes assume a faster trajectory to healthier fat indicating a quantitative regulatory effect.
A similar pattern is obtained when a model is constructed based on the slow induction of SCD.

DISCUSSION

The history of Japanese Wagyu or "Kobe" beef is intriguing. According to legend,[3]Wagyu cattle were used for heavy burden although fed only rice husks, suggesting that they may have been selected for efficient food conversion combined with an ability to utilise fatty acids as a direct energy source.

Much later, after the eating of meat was permitted, selection (according to the Shogun's preferences) must have led to enhanced flavour as found with fine marbling and low melting temperature intramuscular fat. Another consequence has been a tendency to muscle weakness attributed to the replacement of myocytes with adipocytes. Whatever the selection criteria, Wagyu have conserved the capacity to marble from their remote North Asian ancestors and seemingly still do so after crossing with diverse breeds now found world-wide. This history suggested that there must be highly conserved and penetrant haplotypes rather than recent random mutations.

The present study began with the seemingly simple aim of improving the healthiness of beef by crossing elite Japanese Wagyu with composite breeds able to survive in harsh conditions. The literature suggests that transfer of a Wagyu gene might improve the fat content thereby providing cholesterol lowering, statin-sparing, tasty beef at reasonable cost. Experience has shown that improvement can occur but inconsistently and only after expensive grain-feeding thereby restricting world-wide access to potential benefits. Our interpretation is that the outcome depends on the particular mix of conserved haplotypes which exert quantitative control over all the multiple functions which shift the balance from muscle to lipid and especially MUFA.

As shown elsewhere,[60] it was necessary to develop a simple method of measuring the amount of beneficial fat. It transpires that heritability of the preferred fat can be demonstrated with T_m but not the standard visual method of quantifying marbling. Hitherto, therefore, selection of sires must have suffered. This is important because, using T_m, the sire effect is evident within one generation meaning that success or failure can occur rapidly, leading to the remarkable scatter as demonstrated in Figure 2. Fortunately, T_m measurements should lead to progressive improvement.

Given accurate and precise measurement of the endpoints, we have used three datasets.

Samples from a tasting competition reveal that some crossbreds can be as desirable as the most elite Wagyu. Here, we offer a strategy based on the observation that transmission of a certain Wagyu haplotype, such as 60.10.S.10, may dramatically improve quality. If confirmed, a homozygous bull will benefit all progeny and remove some of the existing inconsistency and expense. In an ongoing multi-centre study, we hope to be able to evaluate the benefits of sires which are homozygous for 30.20.S.20 and 60.10.S.10 in their anticipated order of benefit. However, because of relatively low haplotype frequencies of say 0.05, the natural frequencies of homozygotes will be less than 0.0025 meaning that the value of such homozygotes will only be clear if all bulls are haplotyped. The solution to the lack of homozygotes for use today is being addressed through Artificial Insemination and Embryo Transfer. In the meanwhile, we are developing some hypotheses which recognize that evaluating all combinations of multi-megabase haplotypes (as diplotypes) is impractical. The *n* values required for the comparisons are greater than the number of cattle alive today.

One of these hypotheses arose from the ability to compare two totally different datasets. The Mayura set standardizes essentially all variables, other than the within Wagyu genetics. The Melaleuka set uses T_m /DOF as a measure to compare crossbreds.

Both show a remarkable effect of TCAP 10,10 v 20,20. It should be emphasized that differences at TCAP itself cannot explain all findings such as the superiority of Wagyu over other breeds and the benefit of 60.10.S.10 in crossbreds.

Rather, taken together the results argue for the importance of ancestral haplotypes rather than individual loci. This is illustrated in Figure 4. The alleles at GH and FASN are different depending upon the megabase haplotype, meaning that effects attributed to these individual alleles could reflect sequences more than 10 megabases away. Therefore, it is important to define the megabase haplotypes before sequencing or SNP analyses. No doubt, this explains why progress has been slow. Genomic analysis of polygenic traits like QTLs must consider the implications of synteny and the potential importance of paralogy, duplication, copy number, retroviral regulators to list a few mechanisms.[2,3,30,31,55] As proposed here, duplication and copy number are more relevant than coding region differences. So too is regulation over extensive distances. Thus SREBF1 is a master regulator which controls gene expression within the SREBF1 to FASN region via targeting transcriptional repressors of MPRIP, TCAP and other muscle–related genes (BECN1, CACNB1, MYH2, MYH3, MYH13); one of these repressors BHLHB 2 maps near FASN.[55] Note also that Muscular dystrophy, limb girdle type 2G is associated in humans with TCAP polymorphism (OMIM#604488) and the histopathology resembles marbling in some respects. Lipid accumulation has been observed in limb girdle muscular dystrophy.[61] Another unexpected recent finding is the location of UTS2R which is associated with development of type II diabetes and fat deposition.[44]

The balance between myogenesis and adipogenesis may be regulated in part by the TCAP - Myostatin pathway in Wagyu as first suggested by Shibata et al. 2006.

We conclude that genomic differences regulate the amount of MUFA such as Oleic Acid in beef and determine the *rate* at which T_m falls with DOF. We regard this finding as indicating, possibly for the first time in the setting of genomics, that the genetic dissection confirms the expectation that the important differences are conserved and quantitative, rather than qualitative, in keeping with our earlier studies on regulation of immunoglobulin and antibodies by MHC ancestral haplotypes.[2,11–13]

Genomic markers for favorable rates of marbling will be of practical as well as theoretical interest. Reducing the time and cost on feed brings the potential to provide healthy beef to a wider sector of the world's population with the secondary benefits of reducing cardiovascular disease and the billions of dollars spent on cholesterol lowering statins.

One of the most important lessons from the present study is that a haplotype sequence of multiple genes and regulators can have complex associations and confounding effects. The 60.10.S.10 haplotypes are Wagyu specific, beneficial in upgrading non-Wagyu in the tasting competition, directly or indirectly associated with low T_m but only the 3rd or 4th best in the ranking of the Wagyu haplotypes. We believe that further data will show that, as in the case of the human MHC, diplotypes and their quantitative *cis* and *trans* interactions will be critical in explaining apparent contradictions.

In conclusion, we recommend combining an accurate measurement of the phenotype with a genomic description of the genotype allowing identification of megabase ancestral haplotypes.

MATERIALS AND METHODS

Full-blood Wagyu with Identified Sires

Two cohorts of Wagyu steers (n=128) and heifers (n=6) were fed for approximately 300±20 days on a proprietary ration within a commercial feedlot. One gram samples of meat and intra muscular fat were taken from each carcass from between the 10th and 11th rib. AUS-MEAT marbling score (MS) was scored between the 10th and 11th rib, with an average of 7.6 and a range from 2 to 11. Steers chosen for the sire comparison had their paternity confirmed via DNA testing.[55]

Branded Beef Competition

Samples were obtained from 9 full blood, 16 crossbred and 4 grass fed entries to the Australian Wagyu Association's "Branded Beef Competition" from 2014 and 2015. Crossbred entries were F1, F2, F3 and F4 Wagyu. Feed composition and days on feed varied but all entries had more than 25% intramuscular fat, as assessed by camera image analysis.[65]

Short-Fed European and crossbreds

The herd at Melaleuka Stud has a variety of European breeds including Simmental, Gelbvieh and Angus. This herd was selected to produce high quality beef on pasture, finished with 2 to 4 months of supplemental feeding. Black Wagyu have been introduced into the herd as full blood or pure bred and for crossing with some of the European breeds. Those designated 50% are the F1 progeny of a mating between Wagyu and European, whereas 25% and 75% are the second cross progeny of F1s mated with European and Wagyu respectively

Akaushi sires have recently been used over some European breed cows with European breed bulls continuing to be used over the remaining cows.

Calves stay on milk until 4 months of age when they are weaned and male calves are castrated. After weaning, they continue grazing Kikuyu and Ryegrass pasture until they reach 300 kg. Their feed is then supplemented with 9 mm EasyBeef pellets (Milne Feeds, Perth, Australia) *ad libitum.* The main ingredients of the EasyBeef pellets are lupins, barley, oats, wheat and triticale. The nutritional composition, based on dry matter, is: Crude Protein (min) 14.5%, Metabolizable Energy (est.) 11.0 MJ/kg., Crude Fiber (max) 20.0%, Urea (max) 1.5%, Monensin 26.6ppm.

The feeders are considered ready for slaughter when they reach a weight of 400kg and are slaughtered to match demand.

Some animals were kept on feed longer to test the effect of increased feeding on T_m and meat quality. The average live weight at slaughter for animals in this study was 461kg, average age at slaughter was 15.4 months (range 8 to 23) and the average days on feed was 104 days (range 17 to 288). Body numbers from abattoirs were matched to farm records and pedigrees via their RFID tags. Where possible identity was confirmed by in-house proprietary DNA testing[40].
Subcutaneous fat samples from the sirloin of these cattle were collected after boning and wet aging.

Long Fed Wagyu Cross breeds with bos indicus ancestry

Fifty samples of subcutaneous fat taken from the rump of crossbred wagyu steers fed for 450 days in a commercial feedlot. Samples were collected from the abattoir and frozen immediately. DNA was extracted and tested for MRIP markers, triglycerides which separated from the adipose tissue during DNA extraction were tested for Tm. Wagyu ancestry ranged from 48% to 96% with the majority being F1 and average Wagyu ancestry at 57%. 19 of the 50 animals had some Bos indicus content. Other dam breeds included Shorthorn and Angus.

DNA extraction and C19 haplotype testing

Genomic DNA was extracted from all meat samples using the standard salting out method. Alleles of SREB, NT5M, MPRIP, TCAP and GH markers were determined by PCR and capillary electrophoresis using the primers and method described in Williamson *et al.* 2011.[55] Alleles of FASN were determined using the primer and method described in Lloyd *et al.* 2013.[56] The FASN marker is more correctly known as SCT-FSN since the present marker is adjacent to the coding region for FASN, within the segmental duplication containing SECTM1. Haplotypes in heterozygous individuals was determined from segregation or alleles in related animals. The W plots were based on haplotype frequencies measured in Australian herds of registered Wagyu.

Acknowledgements

This research was supported by the C Y O'Connor ERADE Village Foundation. The authors would like to thank J.R. Dawkins and the Australian Wagyu Association for samples and associated data. For beef and fat samples we would also like to thank Scott de Bruin (Mayura Station, SA), Peter Gilmour (Irongate Wagyu, WA), Darren Hamblin (Strathdale Wagyu) and Dom Bayard (Global Reproductive Solutions, Goorambatt, VIC). We would like to thank Prof Frank Mastaglia and Sue Lester for their helpful comments.

Contributions

RLD and SSL conceived the paper's outline, the data collection and writing plan. RLD wrote the paper. SSL, EJS and RLD contributed to analysis and correction of the various manuscript versions. EJS was also responsible for the review of the literature summarized in Table 1. JV contributed samples from Melaleuka Stud.

Conflict of Interest

Collectively, the authors associated with the C.Y. O'Connor ERADE Village Foundation
have an interest in the work described in this manuscript as it forms part of the Foundation's intellectual property.

References

[1] S.S. Lloyd, E.J. Steele, R.L. Dawkins, Analysis of Haplotype Sequences, in: J.K. Kulski (Ed.), Next Gener. Seq. - Adv. Appl. Challenges, InTech, 2016: pp. 345–368. doi:10.5772/60489.

[2] R. Dawkins, C. Leelayuwat, S. Gaudieri, G. Tay, J. Hui, S. Cattley, P. Martinez, J. Kulski, Genomics of the major histocompatibility complex: haplotypes, duplication, retroviruses and disease, Immunol. Rev. 167 (1999) 275–304. doi:10.1111/j.1600-065X.1999.tb01399.x.

[3] R.L. Dawkins, Adapting Genetics, Near Urban Publishing, Dallas, TX, 2015.

[4] Z.L. Awdeh, D. Raum, E.J. Yunis, C. a Alper, Extended HLA/complement allele haplotypes: evidence for T/t-like complex in man., Proc. Natl. Acad. Sci. U. S. A. 80 (1983) 259–63.

[5] E.J. Yunis, C.E. Larsen, M. Fernandez-Vina, Z.L. Awdeh, T. Romero, J.A. Hansen, C.A. Alper, Inheritable variable sizes of DNA stretches in the human MHC: conserved extended haplotypes and their fragments or blocks, Tissue Antigens. 62 (2003) 1–20. doi:098 [pii].

[6] C.A. Alper, D. Marcus-Bagley, Z. Awdeh, M.S. Kruskall, G.S. Eisenbarth, S.J. Brink, A.J. Katz, R. Stein, D.H. Bing, E.J. Yunis, P.H. Schur, Prospective analysis suggests susceptibility genes for deficiency of IgA and several other immunoglobulins on the [HLA-B8, SC01, DR3] conserved extended haplotype, Tissue Antigens. 56 (2000) 207–216.

[7] P. Raj, E. Rai, R. Song, S. Khan, B.E. Wakeland, K. Viswanathan, C. Arana, C. Liang, B. Zhang, I. Dozmorov, F. Carr-johnson, M. Mitrovic, G.B. Wiley, J.A. Kelly, B.R. Lauwerys, N.J. Olsen, C. Cotsapas, C.K. Garcia, C.A. Wise, J.B. Harley, S.K. Nath, J.A. James, C.O. Jacob, B.P. Tsao, C. Pasare, D.R. Karp, Q.Z. Li, P.M. Gaffney, E.K. Wakeland, Regulatory polymorphisms modulate the expression of HLA class II molecules and promote autoimmunity, Elife. 5 (2016) e12089. doi:10.7554/eLife.12089.

[8] K.M. Steinberg, F. Antonacci, P.H. Sudmant, J.M. Kidd, C.D. Campbell, L. Vives, M. Malig, L. Scheinfeldt, W. Beggs, M. Ibrahim, G. Lema, T.B. Nyambo, S. a Omar, J.-M. Bodo, A. Froment, M.P. Donnelly, K.K. Kidd, S. a Tishkoff, E.E. Eichler, Structural diversity and African origin of the 17q21.31 inversion polymorphism, Nat. Genet. 44 (2012) 872–880. doi:10.1038/ng.2335.
[9] C.A. Alper, C.E. Larsen, D.P. Dubey, Z.L. Awdeh, D.A. Fici, E.J. Yunis, The haplotype structure of the human major histocompatibility complex, Hum. Immunol. 67 (2006) 73–84. doi:S0198-8859(05)00458-1 [pii] 10.1016/j.humimm.2005.11.006.
[10] G.C. Johnson, L. Esposito, B.J. Barratt, a N. Smith, J. Heward, G. Di Genova, H. Ueda, H.J. Cordell, I. a Eaves, F. Dudbridge, R.C. Twells, F. Payne, W. Hughes, S. Nutland, H. Stevens, P. Carr, E. Tuomilehto-Wolf, J. Tuomilehto, S.C. Gough, D.G. Clayton, J. a Todd, Haplotype tagging for the identification of common disease genes., Nat. Genet. 29 (2001) 233–237. doi:10.1038/ng1001-233.
[11] A.N. Wilton, T.J. Cobain, R.L. Dawkins, Family studies of IgA deficiency, Immunogenetics. 21 (1985) 333–342.
[12] T. Cobain, M. French, F. Christiansen, R. Dawkins, Association of IgA deficiency with HLA A28 and B14, Tissue Antigens. 22 (1983) 151–154.
[13] M.A. French, R.L. Dawkins, Central MHC genes, IgA deficiency and autoimmune disease., Immunol. Today. 11 (1990) 271–274.
[14] H. Sekine, R.C. Ferreira, Q. Pan-Hammarström, R.R. Graham, B. Ziemba, S.S. de Vries, J. Liu, K. Hippen, T. Koeuth, W. Ortmann, A. Iwahori, M.K. Elliott, S. Offer, C. Skon, L. Du, J. Novitzke, A.T. Lee, N. Zhao, J.D. Tompkins, D. Altshuler, P.K. Gregersen, C. Cunningham-Rundles, R.S. Harris, C. Her, D.L. Nelson, L. Hammarström, G.S. Gilkeson, T.W. Behrens, Role for Msh5 in the regulation of Ig class switch recombination., Proc. Natl. Acad. Sci. U. S. A. 104 (2007) 7193–7198. doi:10.1073/pnas.0700815104.
[15] H. Khatib, Molecular and Quantitative Animal Genetics, Wiley-Blackwell, 2015.
[16] G. Simm, Genetic Improvement in Cattle and Sheep, Farming Press - Miller Freeman UK Ltd, Tonbridge, UK, 1998.
[17] W.G. Hill, Applications of population genetics to animal breeding, from wright, fisher and lush to genomic prediction, Genetics. 196 (2014) 1–16. doi:10.1534/genetics.112.147850.
[18] J. Fadista, B. Thomsen, L.-E. Holm, C. Bendixen, Copy number variation in the bovine genome., BMC Genomics. 11 (2010) 284. doi:10.1186/1471-2164-11-284.
[19] Y. Hou, D.M. Bickhart, M.L. Hvinden, C. Li, J. Song, D. a Boichard, S. Fritz, A. Eggen, S. DeNise, G.R. Wiggans, T.S. Sonstegard, C.P. Van Tassell, G.E. Liu, Fine mapping of copy number variations on two cattle genome assemblies using high density SNP array, BMC Genomics. 13 (2012) 376. doi:10.1186/1471-2164-13-376.
[20] Y. Hou, G.E. Liu, D.M. Bickhart, M.F. Cardone, K. Wang, E.-S. Kim, L.K. Matukumalli, M. Ventura, J. Song, P.M. VanRaden, T.S. Sonstegard, C.P. Van Tassell, Genomic characteristics of cattle copy number variations., BMC Genomics. 12 (2011) 127. doi:10.1186/1471-2164-12-127.

[21] D.M. Bickhart, Y. Hou, S.G. Schroeder, C. Alkan, M.F. Cardone, L.K. Matukumalli, J. Song, R.D. Schnabel, M. Ventura, J.F. Taylor, J.F. Garcia, C.P. Van Tassell, T.S. Sonstegard, E.E. Eichler, G.E. Liu, Copy number variation of individual cattle genomes using next-generation sequencing, Genome Res. 22 (2012) 778–790. doi:10.1101/gr.133967.111.
[22] L. Fontanesi, F. Beretti, P.L. Martelli, M. Colombo, S. Dall'Olio, M. Occidente, B. Portolano, R. Casadio, D. Matassino, V. Russo, A first comparative map of copy number variations in the sheep genome, Genomics. 97 (2011) 158–165. doi:10.1016/j.ygeno.2010.11.005.
[23] J. Liu, L. Zhang, L. Xu, H. Ren, J. Lu, X. Zhang, S. Zhang, X. Zhou, C. Wei, F. Zhao, L. Du, Analysis of copy number variations in the sheep genome using 50K SNP BeadChip array., BMC Genomics. 14 (2013) 229. doi:10.1186/1471-2164-14-229.
[24] P.U. Cameron, H.A. Tabarias, B. Pulendran, W. Robinson, R.L. Dawkins, Conservation of the central MHC genome: PFGE mapping and RFLP analysis of complement, HSP70, and TNF genes in the goat., Immunogenetics. 31 (1990) 253–264. doi:10.1007/BF00204897.
[25] C.A. McLure, P.W. Kesners, S. Lester, D. Male, C. Amadou, J.R. Dawkins, B.J. Stewart, J.F. Williamson, R.L. Dawkins, Haplotyping of the canine MHC without the need for DLA typing, Int J Immunogenet. 32 (2005) 407–411. doi:EJI549 [pii] 10.1111/j.1744-313X.2005.00549.x.
[26] C.E. Alvarez, J.M. Akey, Copy number variation in the domestic dog., Mamm. Genome. 23 (2012) 144–63. doi:10.1007/s00335-011-9369-8.
[27] M.E.O. Locke, M. Milojevic, S.T. Eitutis, N. Patel, A.E. Wishart, M. Daley, K.A. Hill, Genomic copy number variation in Mus musculus, BMC Genomics. 16 (2015) 497. doi:10.1186/s12864-015-1713-z.
[28] J. Wang, J. Jiang, W. Fu, L. Jiang, X. Ding, J.-F. Liu, Q. Zhang, A genome-wide detection of copy number variations using SNP genotyping arrays in swine, BMC Genomics. 13 (2012) 273. doi:10.1186/1471-2164-13-273.
[29] J. Fadista, M. Nygaard, L.-E. Holm, B. Thomsen, C. Bendixen, A snapshot of CNVs in the pig genome., PLoS One. 3 (2008) e3916. doi:10.1371/journal.pone.0003916.
[30] T. Shiina, H. Inoko, J.K. Kulski, An update of the HLA genomic region, locus information and disease associations: 2004, Tissue Antigens. 64 (2004) 631–649. doi:TAN327 [pii] 10.1111/j.1399-0039.2004.00327.x.
[31] C.A. McLure, P. Hinchliffe, S. Lester, J.F. Williamson, J.A. Millman, P.J. Keating, B.J. Stewart, R.L. Dawkins, Genomic Evolution and Polymorphism: Segmental Duplications and Haplotypes at 108 Regions on 21 Chromosomes, Genomics. 102 (2013) 15–26. doi:10.1016/j.ygeno.2013.02.011.
[32] N. Teicholz, The scientific report guiding the US dietary guidelines: is it scientific?, BMJ. 351 (2015) h4962. doi:10.1136/bmj.h4962.
[33] N. Teicholz, A Big Fat Surprise, Simon & Schuster, New York, 2014.
[34] S.B. Smith, B.J. Johnson, Marbling : Management of cattle to maximize the deposition of intramuscular adipose tissue, National cattlemen's beef association, Centennial, CO, 2014.
[35] L.A. Gilmore, R.L. Walzem, S.F. Crouse, D.R. Smith, T.H. Adams, V. Vaidyanathan, X. Cao, S.B. Smith, Consumption of high-oleic acid

ground beef increases HDL-cholesterol concentration but both high- and low-oleic acid ground beef decrease HDL particle diameter in normocholesterolemic men., J. Nutr. 141 (2011) 1188–1194. doi:10.3945/jn.110.136085.

[36] T.H. Adams, R.L. Walzem, D.R. Smith, S. Tseng, S.B. Smith, Hamburger high in total, saturated and trans-fatty acids decreases HDL cholesterol and LDL particle diameter, and increases TAG, in mildly hypercholesterolaemic men., Br. J. Nutr. 103 (2010) 91–8. doi:10.1017/S0007114509991516.

[37] V. Lecomte, E. Meugnier, V. Euthine, C. Durand, D. Freyssenet, G. Nemoz, S. Rome, H. Vidal, E. Lefai, A New Role for Sterol Regulatory Element Binding Protein 1 Transcription Factors in the Regulation of Muscle Mass and Muscle Cell Differentiation, Mol. Cell. Biol. 30 (2010) 1182–1198. doi:10.1128/MCB.00690-09.

[38] A. Ishii, K. Yamaji, Y. Uemoto, N. Sasago, E. Kobayashi, N. Kobayashi, T. Matsuhashi, S. Maruyama, H. Matsumoto, S. Sasazaki, H. Mannen, Genome-wide association study for fatty acid composition in Japanese Black cattle., Anim. Sci. J. (2013). doi:10.1111/asj.12063.

[39] Y. Uemoto, T. Abe, N. Tameoka, H. Hasebe, K. Inoue, H. Nakajima, N. Shoji, M. Kobayashi, E. Kobayashi, Whole-genome association study for fatty acid composition of oleic acid in Japanese Black cattle, Anim. Genet. 42 (2011) 141–148. doi:10.1111/j.1365-2052.2010.02088.x.

[40] J.F. Williamson, E.J. Steele, S. Lester, O. Kalai, J.A. Millman, L. Wolrige, D. Bayard, C. McLure, R.L. Dawkins, Genomic evolution in domestic cattle: Ancestral haplotypes and healthy beef, Genomics. 97 (2011) 304–312. doi:S0888-7543(11)00037-1 [pii] 10.1016/j.ygeno.2011.02.006.

[41] S.S. Lloyd, D. Bayard, S. Lester, J.F. Williamson, E.J. Steele, R.L. Dawkins, Ancestral Haplotypes, Quantal Genomics and Healthy Beef S., in: Proceedings, 10th World Congr. Genet. Appl. to Livest. Prod. Ancestral, 2014.

[42] S.S. Lloyd, D. Bayard, S.A. Lester, J.F. Williamson, R.L. Dawkins, The Value of Haplotyping, INTERBULL Bull. 47 (2013) 252–255.

[43] S.B. Smith, C.A. Gill, D.K. Lunt, M.A. Brooks, Regulation of Fat and Fatty Acid Composition in Beef Cattle, Asian-Aust. J. Anim. Sci. 22 (2009) 1225–1233.

[44] S.S. Lloyd, S.T. Dawkins, R.L. Dawkins, A novel method of measuring the melting point of animal fats, J. Anim. Sci. 92 (2014) 4775–4778. doi:10.2527/jas.2014-7981.

[45] S.S. Lloyd, J.L. Valenzuela, E.J. Steele, R.L. Dawkins, Genetics of marbling in Wagyu: the value of lipid profiling by melting temperature, International Journal of Genomics. Submitted (2017).

[46] M.D. Grounds, J. Terrill, H. Radley-crabb, T. Robertson, J. Papadimitriou, S. Spuler, T. Shavlakadze, Lipid Accumulation in Dysferlin-Deficient Muscles, Am. J. Pathol. 184 (2014) 1668–1676. doi:10.1016/j.ajpath.2014.02.005.

[47] S. Sasazaki, K. Akiyama, T. Narukami, H. Matsumoto, K. Oyama, H. Mannen, UTS2R gene polymorphisms are associated with fatty acid composition in Japanese beef cattle, Anim. Sci. J. 85 (2014) 499–505. doi:10.1111/asj.12167.

[48] M. Shibata, K. Matsumoto, K. Aikawa, T. Muramoto, S. Fujimura, M. Kadowaki, Gene expression of myostatin during development and

regeneration of skeletal muscle in Japanese Black Cattle, J. Anim. Sci. 84 (2006) 2983–2989. doi:10.2527/jas.2006-118.

[49] J. Krumsiek, R. Arnold, T. Rattei, Gepard: A rapid and sensitive tool for creating dotplots on genome scale, Bioinformatics. 23 (2007) 1026–1028. doi:10.1093/bioinformatics/btm039.

[50] S. Hoashi, N. Ashida, H. Ohsaki, T. Utsugi, S. Sasazaki, M. Taniguchi, K. Oyama, F. Mukai, H. Mannen, Genotype of bovine sterol regulatory element binding protein-1 (SREBP-1) is associated with fatty acid composition in Japanese Black cattle, Mamm Genome. 18 (2007) 880–886. doi:10.1007/s00335-007-9072-y.

[51] M.S.A. Bhuiyan, S.L. Yu, J.T. Jeon, D. Yoon, Y.M. Cho, E.W. Park, N.K. Kim, K.S. Kim, J.H. Lee, DNA Polymorphisms in SREBF1 and FASN Genes Affect Fatty Acid Composition in Korean Cattle (Hanwoo), Asian-Australasian J. Anim. Sci. 22 (2009) 765–773.

[52] T. Matsuhashi, S. Maruyama, Y. Uemoto, N. Kobayashi, H. Mannen, T. Abe, S. Sakaguchi, E. Kobayashi, T. Matsuhashi, S. Maruyama, Y. Uemoto, N. Kobayashi, H. Mannen, Effects of bovine fatty acid synthase, stearoyl-coenzyme A desaturase, sterol regulatory element-binding protein 1, and growth hormone gene polymorphisms on fatty acid composition and carcass traits in Japanese Black cattle., J. Anim. Sci. 89 (2011) 12–22. doi:10.2527/jas.2010-3121.

[53] C. Han, M. Vinsky, N. Aldai, M.E.R. Dugan, T.A. McAllister, C. Li, Association analyses of DNA polymorphisms in bovine SREBP-1, LXRα, FADS1 genes with fatty acid composition in Canadian commercial crossbred beef steers, Meat Sci. 93 (2013) 429–436. doi:10.1016/j.meatsci.2012.10.006.

[54] L. Xu, L.P. Zhang, Z.R. Yuan, L.P. Guo, M. Zhu, X. Gao, H.J. Gao, J.Y. Li, S.Z. Xu, B. Breeding, Polymorphism of SREBP1 is associated with beef fatty acid composition in Simmental bulls, Genet. Mol. Res. 12 (2013) 5802–5809.

[55] H.S. Cheong, D. Yoon, L.H. Kim, B.L. Park, H.W. Lee, C.S. Han, E.M. Kim, H.C. Cho, E.R. Chung, I. Cheong, H.D. Shin, Titin-cap (TCAP) polymorphisms associated with marbling score of beef, Meat Sci. 77 (2007) 257–263. doi:10.1016/j.meatsci.2007.03.014.

[56] A. Ardiyanti, Y. Oki, Y. Suda, K. Suzuki, K. Chikuni, Y. Obara, K. Katoh, Effects of GH gene polymorphism and sex on carcass traits and fatty acid compositions in Japanese Black cattle, Anim Sci J. 80 (2009) 62–69. doi:ASJ594 [pii] 10.1111/j.1740-0929.2008.00594.x.

[57] S. Zhang, T.J. Knight, J.M. Reecy, D.C. Beitz, DNA polymorphisms in bovine fatty acid synthase are associated with beef fatty acid composition, Anim. Genet. 39 (2008) 62–70. doi:10.1111/j.1365-2052.2007.01681.x.

[58] T. Abe, J. Saburi, H. Hasebe, T. Nakagawa, S. Misumi, T. Nade, H. Nakajima, N. Shoji, M. Kobayashi, E. Kobayashi, Novel mutations of the FASN gene and their effect on fatty acid composition in japanese black beef, Biochem. Genet. 47 (2009) 397–411. doi:10.1007/s10528-009-9235-5.

[59] D. Oh, Y. Lee, B. La, J. Yeo, E. Chung, Y. Kim, C. Lee, Fatty acid composition of beef is associated with exonic nucleotide variants of the gene encoding FASN, Mol. Biol. Rep. 39 (2012) 4083–4090. doi:10.1007/s11033-011-1190-7.

[60] M. Saatchi, D.J. Garrick, R.G. Tait, M.S. Mayes, M. Drewnoski, J. Schoonmaker, C. Diaz, D.C. Beitz, J.M. Reecy, Genome-wide association and prediction of direct genomic breeding values for composition of fatty acids in Angus beef cattle., BMC Genomics. 14 (2013) 730. doi:10.1186/1471-2164-14-730.

[61] K. Hayakawa, T. Sakamoto, A. Ishii, K. Yamaji, Y. Uemoto, N. Sasago, E. Kobayashi, N. Kobayashi, T. Matsuhashi, The g.841G>C SNP of FASN gene is associated with fatty acid composition in beef cattle, Anim. Sci. Journal,. 86 (2015) 737–746. doi:10.1111/asj.12357.

[62] L. Bartoň, D. Bureš, T. Kott, D. Řehák, Associations of polymorphisms in bovine DGAT1, FABP4, FASN, and PPARGC1A genes with intramuscular fat content and the fatty acid composition of muscle and subcutaneous fat in Fleckvieh bulls., Meat Sci. 114 (2016) 18–23. doi:10.1016/j.meatsci.2015.12.004.

[63] L. Chen, C. Ekine-Dzivenu, M. Vinsky, J. Basarab, J. Aalhus, M.E.R. Dugan, C. Fitzsimmons, P. Stothard, C. Li, Genome-wide association and genomic prediction of breeding values for fatty acid composition in subcutaneous adipose and longissimus lumborum muscle of beef cattle, BMC Genet. 16 (2015) 135. doi:10.1186/s12863-015-0290-0.

[64] J. Papaleo Mazzucco, D.E.E. Goszczynski, M.V. V. Ripoli, L.M.M. Melucci, A.M.M. Pardo, E. Colatto, A. Rogberg-Muñoz, C.A.A. Mezzadra, G.J.J. Depetris, G. Giovambattista, E.L.L. Villarreal, Growth, carcass and meat quality traits in beef from Angus, Hereford and cross-breed grazing steers, and their association with SNPs in genes related to fat deposition metabolism, Meat Sci. 114 (2016) 121–129. doi:10.1016/j.meatsci.2015.12.018.

[65] K. Kuchida, S. Kono, K. Konishi, L.D. Van Vleck, M. Suzuki, S. Miyoshi, L.D. Van Vleck, Prediction of crude fat content of longissimus muscle of beef using the ratio of fat area calculated from computer image analysis: comparison of regression equations for prediction using different input devices at different stations., J. Anim. Sci. 78 (2000) 799–803.

[66] Y. Iwata, Y. Katanosaka, Y. Arai, M. Shigekawa, S. Wakabayashi, Dominant-negative inhibition of Ca2+ influx via TRPV2 ameliorates muscular dystrophy in animal models, Hum. Mol. Genet. 18 (2009) 824–834. doi:10.1093/hmg/ddn408.

[67] D.J. Lloyd, R.C. Trembath, S. Shackleton, A novel interaction between lamin A and SREBP1: implications for partial lipodystrophy and other laminopathies, Hum. Mol. Genet. 11 (2002) 769–778.

[68] E.S. Moreira, T.J. Wiltshire, G. Faulkner, A. Nilforoushan, M. Vainzof, O.T. Suzuki, G. Valle, R. Reeves, M. Zatz, M.R. Passos-Bueno, D.E. Jenne, Limb-girdle muscular dystrophy type 2G is caused by mutations in the gene encoding the sarcomeric protein telethonin., Nat. Genet. 24 (2000) 163–166. doi:10.1038/72822.

[69] Y.K. Hayashi, C. Matsuda, M. Ogawa, K. Goto, K. Tominaga, S. Mitsuhashi, Y.E. Park, I. Nonaka, N. Hino-Fukuyo, K. Haginoya, H. Sugano, I. Nishino, Human PTRF mutations cause secondary deficiency of caveolins resulting in muscular dystrophy with generalized lipodystrophy, J. Clin. Invest. 119 (2009) 2623–2633. doi:10.1172/JCI38660.

[70] P. Grumati, L. Coletto, P. Sabatelli, M. Cescon, A. Angelin, E. Bertaggia, B. Blaauw, A. Urciuolo, T. Tiepolo, L. Merlini, N.M.

Maraldi, P. Bernardi, M. Sandri, P. Bonaldo, Autophagy is defective in collagen VI muscular dystrophies, and its reactivation rescues myofiber degeneration., Nat. Med. 16 (2010) 1313–1320. doi:10.1038/nm.2247.
[71] M. Trabelsi, N. Kavian, F. Daoud, V. Commere, N. Deburgrave, C. Beugnet, S. Llense, J.C. Barbot, A. Vasson, J.C. Kaplan, F. Leturcq, J. Chelly, Revised spectrum of mutations in sarcoglycanopathies, Eur J Hum Genet. 16 (2008) 793–803. doi:ejhg20089 [pii]\r10.1038/ejhg.2008.9.

FIGURES AND TABLES

Figure 1: Marbling and Muscular Dystrophy are Syntenic on Bota 19 and Chromosome 17

SREB-BHBLB regulated muscle genes

a	MYH13
b	MYH2
c	MYH3
d	MPRIP
e	SREBF1
f	CACNB1
g	TCAP
h	BECN1
i	ENO3
j	CACNG1

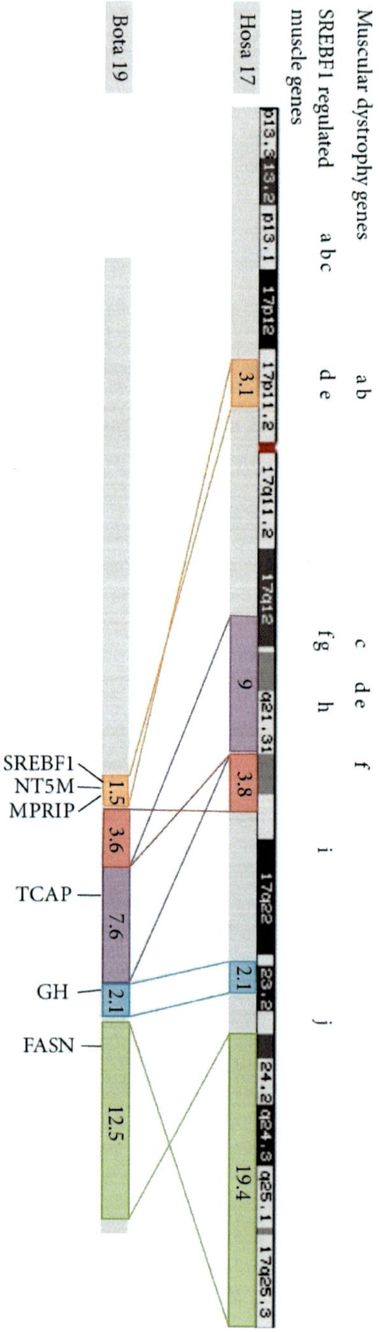

Muscular Dystrophy Genes

a	TRPV2	Muscular dystrophy is ameliorated in dystrophin-deficient mdx mice by dominant-negative inhibition of TRPV2 (Iwata et al. 2009)
b	SREBF1	Mutations of LMNA that cause Emery-Dreifuss muscular dystrophy (EDMD2-AD) and familial partial lipodystrophy (FPLD2) result in less binding of lamin A to SREBP1. (Lloyd et al. 2002)
c	TCAP	Limb-girdle muscular dystrophy type 2G (LGMD2G) is caused by mutations in the TCAP gene (Moreira et al. 2000)
d	PTRF	Congenital generalized lipodystrophy, type 4; (CGL4) is caused by mutations in PTRF that result in CAV 3 deficiency.
e	BECN1	Expression of BECN1 was reduced in patients with muscular dystrophies BTHLM1 and UMCD1 which were caused by COL6A1 mutations.
f	SGCA	Sarcoglycans form part of the dystrophin-glycoprotein complex. Mutations in SGCA cause Limb-girdle muscular dystrophy type 2D (LGMD2D). SGCB, SGCD and SGCG are associated with LGMD types 2E, 2F and 2C respectively. (Trabelsi 2008)

Legend Figure 1: Coloured boxes represent segments with the same gene content. Crossed joining lines indicate inverted translocations. Numbers represent Mb.

Synteny was determined by the positions of homologous genes in the human assembly Hg 38 and Bovine assembly BosTau8 located using the UCSC Genome browser. Inverted sections and the exact location of boundaries between blocks were determined by dotplots[63] comparing the two sequences. The annotated dotplots used are shown in Supplementary Figure 1. The positions of genes associated with muscular dystrophy are shown in the first row of letters above Hosa 17. The association to muscular dystrophy is shown in the table below. The positions of genes involved in the regulation of muscle development by SREBF1, either directly or through BHLHE40 and BHLHE41 (previously known as BHLHB2 and BHLHB3 respectively) are shown in the second row of letters above Hosa 17. Adapted from [3] with permission. We thank Joe Williamson for assistance with this figure.

Figure 2: Polymorphic markers define conserved extended C19 ancestral haplotypes:

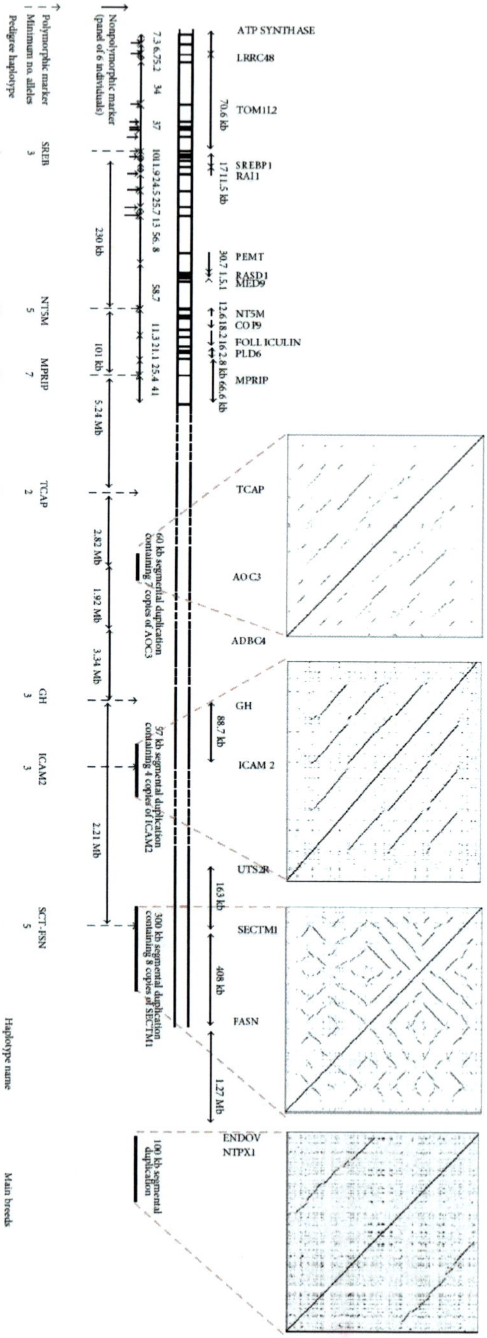

Figure 2: *Polymorphic markers define conserved extended C19 ancestral haplotypes*: This region on BTAchr19 is bounded by markers SREBF1 and FASN (See [56] for details. The FASN marker is more correctly known as SCT-FSN since the present marker is adjacent to the coding region for FASN, within the segmental duplication containing SECTM1. The map positions of PCR markers and the number and type of alleles at each locus are indicated including the main high frequency and largely breed-specific haplotypes extending from SREBF1 to TCAP. We have extended the haplotyping through the region and plan to develop more markers based on the potential polymorphism revealed by the structural duplications extending from 43Mb to 52Mb (Figure and below). Note the regions where PCR product polymorphism was not detected.[56]

Structural duplications in C19 35-55Mb region : We used the current Cow genome assembly (Bos_tauros_UMD_3.1.1/bostau8 Assembly) on the UCSC Web Browser and searched the chr19 region from 35Mb to 55Mb in 500Kb sectors for large structural segmental duplications using standard dot-plotting methods aligning each 500Kb sector against itself (Gepard 1.30).[63] We found clusters of rolling, sometimes clustered-inverted, segmental duplications in the reference genome on chr19 at 43.51 Mb (~60Kb in length), 43.86 Mb (~90Kb), 48.86 (~57Kb) and 50.846Mb (~300Kb). We also found a long single imperfect duplication of 103-112Kb at 52.73Mb and 52.88Mb. Some of these dot plots are shown as cutaways in the Figure. This region has a relatively low density of protein coding genes.

Figure 3: Segregation of 20MB haplotype through three generations of Wagyu Pedigree.

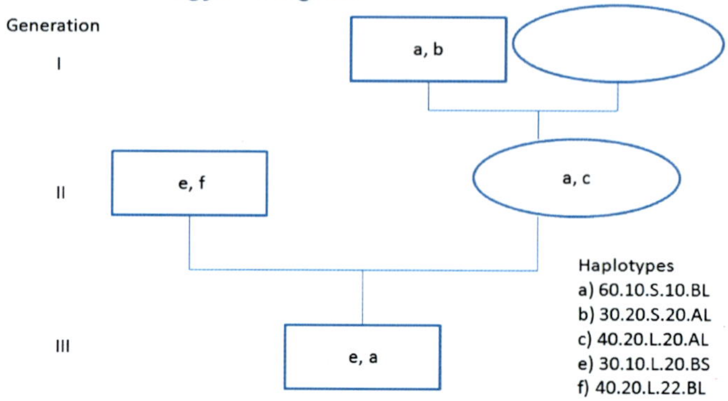

Figure 3: Haplotype *a* is inherited intact from the maternal grandsire. The calf, dam and maternal grandsire are all heterozygous at the SREBF1 or NT5M and GH or FASN markers, which allows the segregation of haplotype *a* to be seen clearly.

Figure 4: W Plot comparing haplotype frequencies in Wagyu and Simmental.

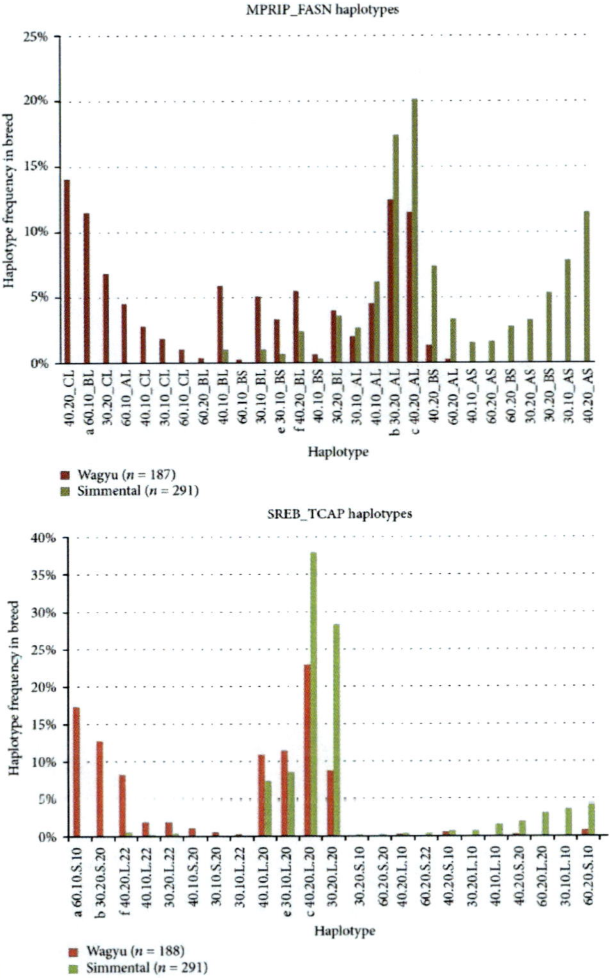

a)

b)

Figure 4: W plot comparing haplotype frequencies in Wagyu and Simmental. Adapted from [58]. (a) The haplotypes are from MPRIP to FASN (see Figure 2). Note SCT-FSN L in Wagyu and S in Simmental, also GH C in Wagyu and GH A in Simmental with GH B largely in the haplotypes common to both breeds. Haplotype designation is MPRIP.TCAP_GH SCT-FSN. (b) Haplotypes are from SREBF1 to TCAP. Haplotype designation is MPRIP.TCAP.SREB.NT5M. The four most common haplotypes of Simmental are also found at high frequency in Wagyu (and many other breeds not shown here), while two of the three most common haplotypes of Wagyu are not found in Simmental (and are not common in any other breed tested).

Figure 5: Crossbreds perform as Wagyu if they possess a Wagyu haplotype

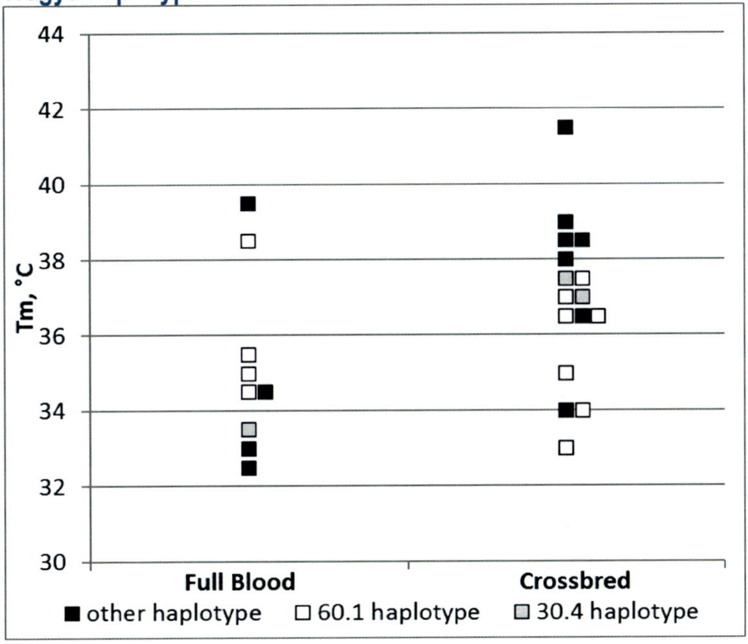

Figure 5: T_m measurements from 9 full blood and 16 crossbred entries to AWA branded beef competition from 2014 and 2015. There are crossbred Wagyu with T_m as low as full bloods. Mean T_m with error bars ±1 SEM. SREB-TCAP haplotypes. White squares indicate animals with at least one 60.10.S.10 haplotype, Pale grey squares indicate animals with at least one 30.20.S.20 haplotype, dark grey squares indicate animals with neither common Wagyu haplotype.

Figure 6: Dot plots of T_m values in Wagyu 300±20 DOF in animals homozygous for the 5.24 Mb region MPRIP-TCAP

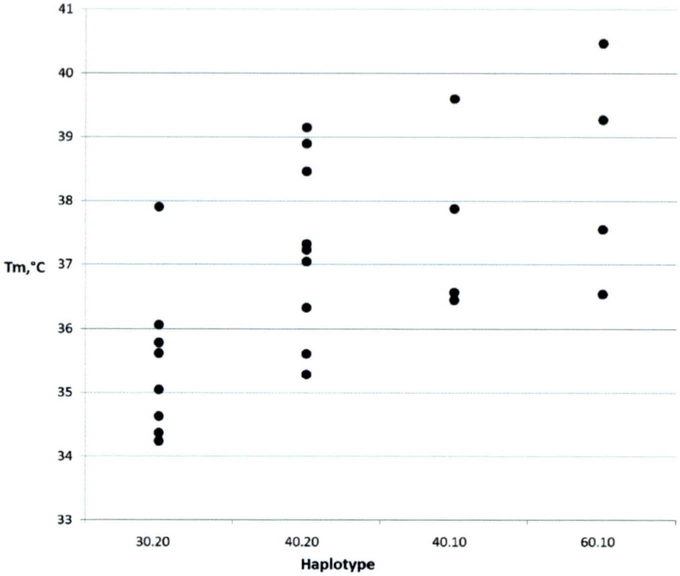

C19 Homozygous Haplotype

Figure 6: Wagyu cattle bred on different Australian farms (Goorambat, Iron Gate Wagyu, Mayura, Rosevale, Peppermint Grove) were fed for 300 days at Mayura Station, South Australia, and beef/fat samples were assayed for C19 haplotypes and fat melting point T_m as indicated in Materials and Methods. Each dot point represents a different homozygote. Homozygous haplotypes for MPRIP-TCAP region only. Students *t-test* for 30.20 v 40.20 yields $P = 0.012$.

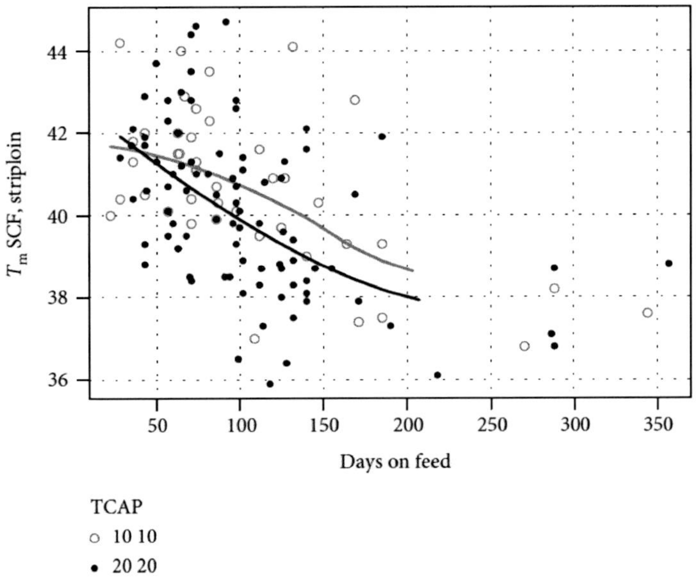

Figure 7. TCAP 20 homozygotes (filled circles) achieve low T_m with less days on feed. Hollow circles show TCAP 10 homozygotes. The smoothed lines were calculated in R with a span of 100. Tm measured on various European and Japanese breeds and crossbreeds including Simmental, Gelbvieh, Black Wagyu, Red Wagyu. Subcutaneous fat samples were taken from the rump and front ends of striploins, with the Tm reported as the average of the two samples. Striploins were DNA tested to confirm a match to the animal sent to abattoir. 42 samples from TCAP 10 homozygotes and 87 samples from TCAP 20 homozygotes are shown. Tm measurements of 105 samples from TCAP 10 20 heterozygotes have been excluded from the graph for simplicity.

Figure 8: TCAP 20 animals have significantly lower Tm for 50-150 days on feed.

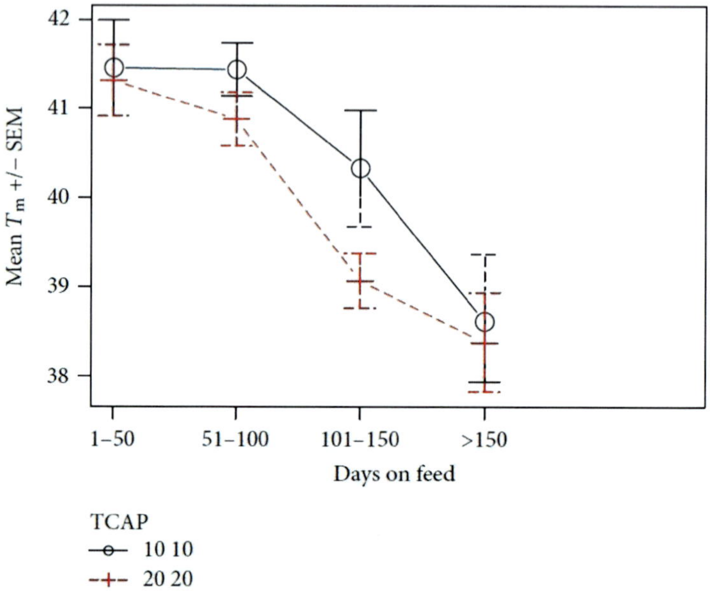

The presence of homozygous 20 TCAP alleles makes the decrease in Tm occur at less days on feed. The initial Tm is similar between the two groups. The Tm in both groups appears to reach a minimum level with long feeding that is not affected by the TCAP allele.

Figure 9: Match to desaturation model of fat melting point

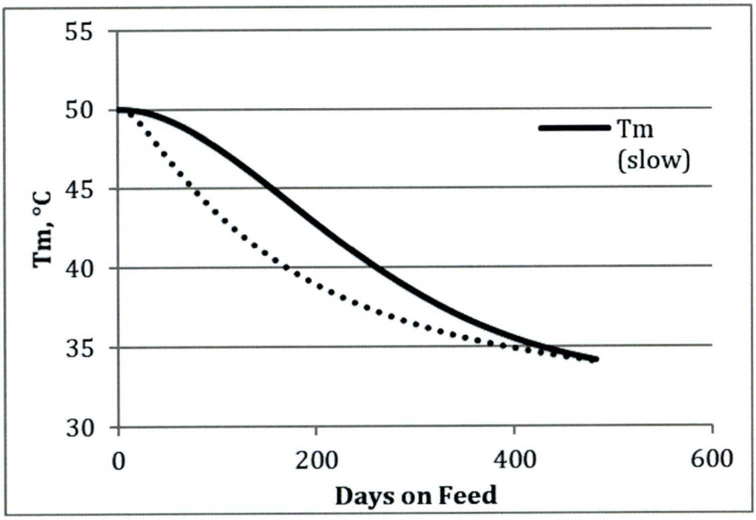

The Tm decrease shown in Figure 7 can be described by the following mathematical model of fat production and desaturation
De novo fat production is controlled by FASN, in response to energy balance. This fat starts saturated. It is then desaturated by the SCD enzyme. The total fat present (F) can be described by dF/d*t* = *a*, where *a* is the rate of de novo fat production. The amount of unsaturated fat (U) increases in proportion to the amount of desaturation enzyme E as: dU/d*t*.= E. In this model the amount of enzyme available is increased in response to the amount of saturated fat present, and also decays. The amount of Enzyme is described by dE/dt = bS – cE, where b and c are constant control parameters and S=F-U is the amount of fat that remains unsaturated. The melting point decreases with increasing proportion of unsaturated fat. T_m decreases in proportion to the amount of unsaturated fat, $T_m = T_\Delta$ S/F $+T_{U.}$
The melting point curves resulting from this model have an initial high Tm decreasing slowly at first, and then more rapidly as the desaturation enzyme builds up. Figure 9 shows how the model reacts to parameter changes. The fast enzyme response with parameters b=.001, c=.1 looks similar to the Tm curve shown in Figure 8 TCAP 20 homozygotes. A slower enzyme response has parameters of b=.0001, c=.01 is more similar to the Tm curve for TCAP 10 homozygotes. TCAP is already known to be involved in pathways regulating the production of the SCD enzyme so it influences the Tm in this way is not surprising.

Table 1: Candidate Genes at c19 35Mb to 55Mb with Reported Associations with Fatty Acid Composition

Gene	Ref	Effect on Intramuscular Fatty Acid Composition in Beef Cattle Muscle Tissues
SREBF1	[50]	In Japanese Black cattle: S allele associated higher MUFA and 1.6°C lower T_m of IMF
	[51]	In Korean Hanwoo cattle: SS alleles IMF stearic acid (C18:0) lower than LL (P<0.05) but linoleic and PUFA contents higher in SS compared to LL (p<0.05).
	[52]	In Japanese Black cattle: No associations with fatty acid composition or meat yield traits
	[53]	Canadian crossbred steers S/L polymorphism associated with 9c C17:1 (P=0.013).
	[54]	Simmental Bulls, Snow Dragon Black: LL higher palmitic acid (C16:1), triglycerides, and C16 index but lower stearic acid (C18:0) and SFA compared with the LS genotype (P < 0.05).
TCAP	[55]	In Korean Hanwoo cattle: a 6 bp Leu-Gln deletion as well as SNP in intron 1 associates with Marbling Score (P=0.02, P=0.003 respectively).
GH	[56]	In Japanese Black cattle: A allele associated low T_m fat; allele B gave higher % C18:1n=9 IMF (P<0.05); allele C gave higher C18:1 MUFA, higher USFA & (P<0.05). Allele C also gave lower % Saturated fatty Acid (SFA), a higher MUFA/SFA ratio and lower T_m of fat (P<0.01).
	[52]	GH L127V polymorphism (A/B Ardiyanti et al 2009) claimed association with IMF fatty acid composition, but not as strong as FASN, SCD or SREBF1
UTS2R	[47]	Japanese Black 7 Holstein cattle: Reported differential association between breeds with marbling and non-synonymous SNP in coding region.
FASN	[57]	Angus bulls: SNP coding region g.17924A>G (as GG genotype) associated FA composition – lower myristic acid (C14:0 P<0.00001), palmitic acid (C16:0 P<0.05) and total saturated FA (P<0.01) in total lipids and TAG than g.17924AA genotype.
	[58]	Japanese Black x Limousin F2 exon 34 SNPs (g.16024A>G (T1950A), g.16039T>C (W1955R). TW changes together increase C18:0, C18:1 content, increase MUFA:SFA ratio.
	[51]	Korean Hanwoo cattle: g17924G>A SNP as GG genotype with higher Oleic Acid (C18:1) palmitic acid (C16:0).
	[39]	GWAS Oleic Acid signal g.16024A>G
	[38]	GWAS reveal significant SNP signals associated FA composition near FASN gene. Confirms Uemoto et al 2011
	[52]	Japanese Black cattle: significant effects on C14:0, C14:1, C18:0, oleic acid C18:1 and MUFA (all P<0.001)
	[59]	Hanwoo Korean cattle: All 5 known exonic SNPs associated with FA composition IMF and Marbling Score
	[60]	Angus cattle: GWAS 51st Mb window on c19 harboring FASN associated with FA composition of IMF
	[61]	Japanese Black cattle: Seven known SNPs. Promoter g.841G>C- improved FA composition IMF
	[62]	Fleckvieh bulls: Known FASN SNPs significant associations C14:0, C16:0, C18:1n-9 in IMF
	[63]	Canadian study: GWAS, same bead chip as Uemoto et al 2011 "markers have large effects near FASN and SCD"
	[64]	Angus,Hereford, Limousin crossbreds: g.16024A>G SNP. AG genotype with higher IMF than GG genotype

SREBF1 - transcription factor that regulates gene expression levels of stearoyl-CoA desaturase (SCD) leading predominantly to mono unsaturated fatty acid (MUFA) Oleic Acid C18:1n=9 in intramuscular fat (IMF); TCAP- Titin-cap or Telethonin, interacts with Titin cap structure and regulates, by inhibition, myostatin hormone secretion; GH1 – growth hormone; UTS2R – urotensin 2 receptor; FASN- Fatty Acid Synthetase

Table 2 Mayura Data 300±20 DOF – 100% Wagyu Associations of Alleles with Low or High T_m

Table 2a

SREBF1 Alleles

T_m	S	L	Total
<37°C	41	89	130
≥37°C	52	82	134
Total	93	171	264

Fisher Exact test statistic 0.25. Not significant at $p<0.05$

Table 2b

NT5M Alleles

T_m	10	20	22	Total
<37°C	19	84	27	130
≥37°C	32	82	20	134
Total	51	166	47	264

Chi-squared statistic is 4.32. The p-value is 0.1. Not significant at $p<0.05$

Table 2c

MPRIP Alleles†

T_m	30	40	60	Total
<37°C	48	60	18	126
≥37°C	34	66	32	132
Total	82	126	50	258

Chi-squared statistic is 6.5. The p-value is 0.04. Result is significant at $p<0.05$

Table 2d

TCAP Alleles

T_m	10	20	Total
<37°C	55	75	130
≥37°C	74	60	134
Total	129	135	264

Fisher Exact test statistic 0.04. Result is significant at $p<0.05$

† The total is lower as some animals with T_m were not typed for MPRIP allele

WAGYU BEEF PRODUCTION IN AUSTRALIA

Sally S Lloyd[1,2,3,] and Roger L Dawkins[1,2,3]
1 CY O'Connor ERADE Village Foundation, PO Box 5100 Canning Vale South, Western Australia, Australia 6155
2 Melaleuka Stud, 24 Genomics Rise, Piara Waters, Western Australia, Australia 6112
3 Centre for Innovation in Agriculture, Murdoch University, Murdoch, Western Australia, Australia 6150 e-mail: slloyd@cyo.edu.au

ABSTRACT

Australian production of Wagyu beef is focused on export markets in Japan and China. For this market marble score and carcass weight determine the price received, and therefore are the primary attributes selected for. Australian production systems make use of available land for grazing. Cows and calves are grazed on pasture with little supplementation until the calves are 4 to 6 months old. In this context, traits for milk, growth and hardiness are also important and can be accessed through cross breeding. Australian consumers are health conscious and beef consumption has been dropping, based on health warnings against its saturated fat content. When purchasing raw beef for home consumption health conscious consumers have chosen lean beef. Red and black Wagyu can be sold in this market at a premium based on a higher proportion of mono unsaturated fats. Melting temperature can be measured easily and is an excellent indicator of the saturated fat ratio and thus the healthiness of beef fat. We have compared fat samples of Various European breeds crossed with Red and Black Wagyu. The beneficial effects of Wagyu ancestry on fatty acid composition are seen at the first cross, even with less than 100 days on feed. Further research will identify specific genetics that support high marbling and low melting point fat within full blood, pure bred and cross bred populations. Production systems also influence fat deposition with myths and secrets surrounding advice on the best diets to optimize marbling. Controlled trials with paired animals, matched for genetics and early growth rate, will shed light on how these feeds effect fat deposition and fatty acid composition.

INTRODUCTION

Australian production of Wagyu beef is focused on export markets in Asia and, for premium product, Japan and China. For this market, marble score and carcass weight determine the price received and are therefore the primary attributes for selection. However, there is no agreed and standardised system for the accurate measurement of marbling.

RESULTS AND DISCUSSION

MEASURING MARBLING

In Australia, an inspector compares the appearance with a card although some Centre's are now also using the KUCHIDA camera.(Kuchida et al., 2000) DEXA scanning is also being assessed. We and some of the leading breeders use the melting temperature of fat,(Lloyd et al., 2014) as discussed below, since the measurement is precise, accurate, genetically determined (Lloyd et al., 2017) and relevant to health as well as taste. To compound the problems for the importer of Australian Wagyu, different scales are used. Therefore, at the present time, marble scores should be used to rank samples from one supplier but should not be the basis of comparisons between different suppliers. Ultimately, each importer, whether of embryos, live or boxed Wagyu, must be guided by consumer preference. Extreme marbling by any measure is in demand in elite settings but modest and even minimal marbling is growing very rapidly based on consumer demand in our own experience. We expect that there will be substantial growth in the demand for lesser degrees of marbling as the consumer becomes more cost and health conscious.

INFLUENCE OF DIFFERENT ENVIRONMENTS

Australian production systems make use of differing landforms for grazing. Cows and calves may be grazed on pasture with little supplementation until the calves are 4 to 6 months old. In this context, traits for milk, growth and hardiness are critically important and are often accessed through cross breeding. In different regions, the cross breeding will be based on the performance of the mother. This is the explanation for the various F1 crosses with Friesian, Angus, Simmental, Shorthorn or, in Northern regions, Bos Indicus sub-breeds such as Santa Gertrudis, Droughtmaster and others. It appears that all cross breeds can marble to various degrees, including Brahman, but the proportion depends on the ancestry of the bull and dam. Some breeders have managed to find the right balance between a hardy, locally adapted mother and a bull which is penetrant with such dams. Our research is addressing such issues. We know (Lloyd et al. in press) that the 60.1 haplotype is penetrant in full- blood and Angus F1s, but there is more to do, and we are willing to support scholarships and fellowships which are relevant to finding the appropriate balances for Asian markets especially if they involve expertise in genomics.

Table 1. Higher Marble Score in F1 and F2 Wagyu with wagyu specific haplotypes compared to bos indicus specific haplotypes.

	Average MS[a]	N	SEM
Bos Indicus Haplotypes[b]	4.2	6	0.54
Wagyu Haplotypes[c]	5.3	22	0.22

[a]Cross bred and pure bred Wagyu fed for 450 days marbling assessed visually between the 10th and 11th rib, using the AUS-Meat marble scale.

[b]Haplotypes classified as Bos Indicus specific were those with MRIP>60 or NT5M>22.

[c]Haplotypes classified as wagyu specific were 60.10.S.10, 30.20.S.20 and 30.10.S.20. Haplotypes were determined for SREB to TCAP markers by a combination of pedigree analysis, homozygosity and breed based haplotype frequencies. For simplicity animals with neither a Bos Indicus specific nor a wagyu specific haplotype have been excluded from the table.

HEALTH

Australian and American consumers are health conscious. Through completion with other species, beef consumption has been dropping based on health warnings against its content of saturated fat. When purchasing raw beef for home consumption health conscious consumers have chosen lean beef. Red and Black Wagyu can be sold in this market at a premium based on a higher proportion of mono unsaturated fats. Melting temperature can be measured easily and is an excellent indicator of the saturated fat ratio and thus the healthiness of beef fat. We have compared fat samples of various European breeds crossed with Red and Black Wagyu. In terms of healthy fatty acid composition, the beneficial effects of Wagyu ancestry are seen at the first cross, even with less than 100 days on feed see Figure 1.

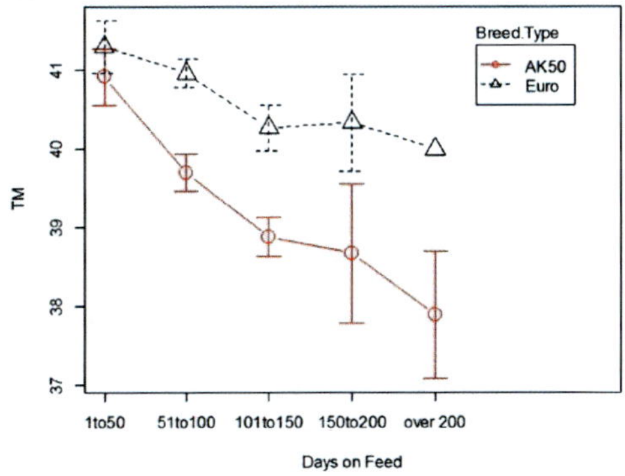

DOF	No. AK50	No. Euro
1-50	5	27
51-100	33	97
101-150	31	34
150-200	5	8
Over 200	2	1

Fig. 1. Tm was measured for subcutaneous fat samples taken from the strip loins of 243 carcasses. The cattle were backgrounded on pasture and then fed on pellets until they reached a satisfactory weight and fatness. The results are grouped by days on feed and by breed of sire (European or Akaushi). The dams of all carcasses were similar European breeds.

FEEDING, CONDITIONS

Further research will identify specific genetics that support marbling and low melting point fat within full blood, pure bred and cross bred populations. Production systems influence fat deposition in keeping with the myths and secrets surrounding advice on how to produce the best diets to optimise marbling. Controlled trials with matched pairs to compare regimes which will produced desired amounts of fat deposition, fatty acid composition and consumer satisfaction. It is highly predictable that battery or lot feeding will become increasingly unacceptable. We have compared different feeding situations and can show that happy cattle grow faster. Whether their melting temperature falls in parallel with their preferred environment is another question to be addressed by a PhD project.

BLACK versus RED/BROWN/AKAUSHI versus HANWOO

These Asian breeds have evolved the ancestral haplotypes which carry the alleles on region of Bota 19 which includes the many genes responsible for marbling and healthy beef (Williamson et al., 2011, Lloyd et al., 2013). We assert this fact without having been able to test Hanwoo and hope that this meeting will lead to the availability of comparisons of the relevant Hanwoo DNA so as to complete the matrix. To date, we have shown that black and red wagyu are distinct breeds (shown in Figure 2) but also similar, no doubt reflecting a common origin from Mongolian/ Hanwoo cattle. The fact that black and red marble implicates the MRIP-TCAP region but the fact that reds do enough on grass suggests that we need to understand the interactions between the different alleles and the environment. We have shown that red F1s can lower Tm quickly and are therefore preferable to blacks. A similar analysis of Red and Black Wagyu compared to Hanwoo would be very exciting for us and, no doubt, of great interest to all of you.

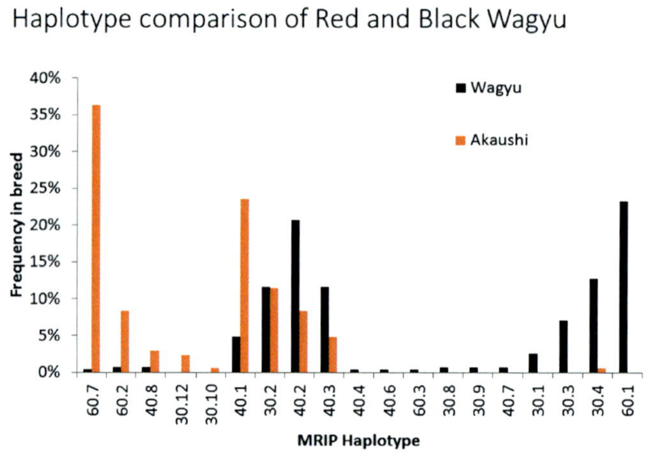

Fig. 2. "W Plot" showing differences in haplotype frequencies between red and black wagyu. The most common haplotypes of red and black wagyu, 60.7 and 60.1 respectively, have similarities in the MRIP – TCAP portion of the haplotype, but differences in the SREB-NT5M end of the haplotype

CONCLUSION

There are many questions remaining on the interactions between breed, haplotypes and optimal feeding conditions. These are best addressed after defining the consumers' preference. To that end, we recommend offering a range of marbling or, in terms of melting temperature, choices between 33 and 38 Celsius.

ACKNOWLEDGEMENTS

Thank you for giving me this opportunity to meet you all and to forge new collaborations. I can send copies of our papers if you contact me on slloyd@cyo.edu.au We, at CYOEVF, thank our collaborators Dom Bayard, Keith Hammond, Scott de Bruin, Darren Hamblin, Peter Hughes, Bruce Cheung, Peter Gilmour and many others for contributing DNA and ideas. Thanks also to JF Williamson, S Lester and H Rebhan.

REFERENCES

Kuchida, K., S. Kono, K. Konishi, L. D. Van Vleck, M. Suzuki, S. Miyoshi & L. D. Van Vleck, 2000. Prediction of crude fat content of longissimus muscle of beef using the ratio of fat area calculated from computer image analysis: comparison of regression equations for prediction using different input devices at different stations. Journal of Animal Science, 78: 799–803.

Lloyd, S. S., D. Bayard, S. A. Lester, J. F. Williamson & R. L. Dawkins, 2013. The Value of Haplotyping. INTERBULL BULLETIN, 47: 252–255.

Lloyd, S. S., S. T. Dawkins & R. L. Dawkins, 2014. A novel method of measuring the melting point of animal fats. Journal of animal science.

Lloyd, S. S., E. J. Steele, J. L. Valenzuela & R. L. Dawkins, 2017. Haplotypes for Type, Degree and Rate of Marbling in Cattle are Syntenic with Human Muscular Dystrophy. International Journal of Genomics, In Press.

Williamson, J. F., E. J. Steele, S. Lester, O. Kalai, J. A. Millman, L. Wolrige, D. Bayard, C. McLure & R. L. Dawkins, 2011. Genomic evolution in domestic cattle: Ancestral haplotypes and healthy beef. Genomics, 97: 304–312.

ADAR deaminase A-to-I editing of DNA and RNA moieties of RNA: DNA hybrids has implications for the mechanism of Ig somatic hypermutation.

Edward J. Steele[a,□], Robyn A. Lindley[b,c]
a CY O'Connor ERADE Village Foundation Inc., Piara Waters, WA, Australia
b GMDxCo Pty Ltd., Hawthorn Vic, Australia
c Department of Pathology, Faculty of Medicine, Dentistry & Health Sciences, University of Melbourne Vic, Australia

Published in DNA Repair, Volume 55, July 2017, Pages 1-6

ABSTRACT

The implications are discussed of recently published biochemical studies on ADAR-mediated A-to-I DNA and RNA deamination at RNA:DNA hybrids. The significance of these data is related to previous work on strand biased and codon-context mutation signatures in B lymphocytes and cancer genomes. Those studies have established that there are two significant strand biases at A:T and G:C base pairs, A-site mutations exceed T-site mutations (A >> T) by 2.9 fold and G-site mutations exceed C-site mutations (G >> C) by 1.7 fold. Both these strand biases are inconsistent with alternative "DNA Deamination" mechanisms, yet are expected consequences of the RNA/RT-based "Reverse Transcriptase" mechanism of immunoglobulin (Ig) somatic hypermutation (SHM). The A-to-I DNA editing component at RNA:DNA hybrids that is likely to occur in Transcription Bubbles, while important, is of far lower A-to-I editing efficiency than in dsRNA substrates. The

RNA moiety of RNA:DNA hybrids is also edited at similar lower frequencies relative to the editing rate at dsRNA substrates. Further, if the A-to-I DNA editing at RNA:DNA hybrids were the sole cause of A-to-I (read as A-to-G) mutation events for Ig SHM in vivo then the exact opposite strand biases at A:T base pairs (T > > A) of what is actually observed (A > > T) would be predicted. It is concluded that the strand-biased somatic mutation patterns at both A:T and G:C base pairs in vivo are best interpreted by the sequential steps of the RNA/RT-based mechanism. Further, the direct DNA A-to-I deamination at Transcription Bubbles is expected to

contribute to the T-to-C component of the strand-biased Ig SHM spectrum.
Full article available from:
https://www.sciencedirect.com/science/article/pii/S1568786417300381

Reverse Transcriptase Mechanism of Somatic Hypermutation: 60 Years of Clonal Selection Theory

Edward J. Steele*

CYO'Connor ERADE Village Foundation Inc., Piara Waters, WA, Australia

Published in Frontiers in Immunology: 23 November 2017

The evidence for the reverse transcriptase mechanism of somatic hypermutation is substantial and multifactorial. In this 60th anniversary year of the publication of Sir MacFarlane Burnet's Clonal Selection Theory, the evidence is briefly reviewed and updated.

Overview
The molecular mechanism underlying somatic hypermutation (SHM) of rearranged immunoglobulin (Ig) genes (V[D]J) has been controversial for some time. Although the process of DNA deamination has dominated discussion in recent years, insufficient attention has been paid to a mechanism based on reverse transcription. One reason therefore for writing this *Perspective* is to counter balance a widely held view in the Ig SHM field that all relevant studies on the molecular mechanism deal only with the "DNA Deamination Model" which ended in complete consensus over 10 years ago sometime between 2004 and 2007 [Table 1 and Ref. (1) in particular]. The other is a personal tribute, in this anniversary year, to the founder of modern immunology, Sir Macfarlane Burnet. It is now 60 years since the publication of the first iteration of "The Clonal Selection Theory of Acquired Immunity" (2), the foundation stone of modern immunology. It was fully expounded in his 1959 book (3) where the main idea was clonal antigenic selection from a pre-existing diverse antibody repertoire from which somatic mutations might

emerge as "forbidden" anti-self clones. Joshua Lederberg then gave the concept sharp molecular focus (4) as did Melvin Cohn and colleagues (5–7). Alastair Cunningham's concept of "clonal variation around a theme" placed antigen-driven SHM firmly within the context of expanding B lymphocyte clones (8). Somatic mutation of Ig variable region genes has therefore been part and parcel of Burnet's clonal selection concept since its inception and is central to a rational understanding of immunological diversification, self-tolerance and the emergence of cancer. We now have a very good idea of the molecular mechanism of SHM. I have chosen to fit this scientific progress within 60 key publications since the late 1950s (Table 1). The most plausible central molecular mechanism of Ig SHM, that fits with and explains all the evidence (9–11) is based on "Reverse Transcription" of the base-modified Ig pre-mRNA (Figure 1). That is, error-prone reverse transcription, by DNA Polymerase-η, of the Ig pre-mRNA template intermediate at rearranged V[D]J gene somatic loci. The Ig pre-mRNA encoding the V[D]J region is copied off the transcribed DNA strand carrying prior AID C-to-U deamination lesions (Uracils and Abasic sites), and it also accumulates ADAR-deaminase mediated RNA editing A-to-I modifications. This already base-modified pre-mRNA sequence is then copied back to the B lymphocyte genomic DNA and integrated at the rearranged V[D]J site (concurrent with antigen-mediated selection of Ig receptor bearing B lymphocytes, Centrocytes, in the Germinal Center). This is essentially the "Reverse Transcriptase Mechanism" which Jeff Pollard and I first published 30 years ago (12). The mechanistic steps, many logical, are clearly outlined in Figure 1, which shows that the characteristic A >> T and G >> C strand bias-generating mutagenic activity is firmly focused on the nascent RNA intermediate in the context of the Transcription Bubble (9–11, 13, 14). Recent publications should be consulted for further definitive ADAR A-to-I editing of both RNA and DNA moieties at RNA:DNA hybrids within Transcription Bubbles (11, 14, 15). Not only is it important to understand the correct molecular mechanism of SHM for cancer diagnosis and detection (16, 17) but also to the current efforts to better understand (18, 19) the origin of Ig diversity involving the mechanism of evolution of the sets germline V segments and the long IGHV and IGLV haplotypes in individual human beings ([20], [21]).

Full Article available from:
https://www.frontiersin.org/articles/10.3389/fimmu.2017.01611/full

Cause of Cambrian Explosion - Terrestrial or Cosmic?

Edward J. Steele[a,j,*], Shirwan Al-Mufti[b], Kenneth A. Augustyn[c], Rohana Chandrajith[d], John P. Coghlan[e], S.G. Coulson[b], Sudipto Ghosh[f], Mark Gillman[g], Reginald M. Gorczynski[h], Brig Klyce[b], Godfrey Louis[i], Kithsiri Mahanama[j], Keith R. Oliver [k], Julio Padron [l], Jiangwen Qu [m], John A. Schuster [n], W.E. Smith[o], Duane P. Snyder[b], Julian A. Steele[p], Brent J. Stewart[a], Robert Temple[q], Gensuke Tokoro[o], Christopher A. Tout[r], Alexander Unzicker[s], Milton Wainwright[b,j], Jamie Wallis[b], Daryl H. Wallis[b], Max K. Wallis[b], John Wetherall[t], D.T. Wickramasinghe[u], J.T. Wickramasinghe[b], N. Chandra Wickramasinghe[b, j, o], Yongsheng Liu [v, w]

a CY O'Connor ERADE Village Foundation, Piara Waters, WA, Australia
b Buckingham Centre for Astrobiology, University of Buckingham, UK
c Center for the Physics of Living Organisms, Department of Physics, Michigan Technological University, Michigan, United States
d Department of Geology, University of Peradeniya, Peradeniya, Sri Lanka
e University of Melbourne, Office of the Dean, Faculty Medicine, Dentistry and Health Sciences, 3rd Level, Alan Gilbert Building, Australia
f Metallurgical & Materials Engineering IIT, Kanpur, India
g South African Brain Research Institute, 6 Campbell Street, Waverly, Johannesburg, South Africa
h University Toronto Health Network, Toronto General Hospital, University of Toronto, Canada
i Department of Physics, Cochin University of Science and Technology Cochin, India
j Centre for Astrobiology, University of Ruhuna, Matara, Sri Lanka
k School of Veterinary and Life Sciences Murdoch University, Perth, WA, Australia
l Studio Eutropi, Clinical Pathology and Nutrition, Via Pompei 46, Ardea, 00040, Rome, Italy
m Department of Infectious Disease Control, Tianjin Center for Disease Control and Prevention, China
n School of History and Philosophy of Science, Faculty of Science, University of Sydney, Sydney, Australia
o Institute for the Study of Panspermia and Astrobiology, Gifu, Japan
p Centre for Surface Chemistry and Catalysis, KU Leuven, Celestijnenlaan 200F, 3001, Leuven, Belgium
q The History of Chinese Culture Foundation, Conway Hall, London, UK
r Institute of Astronomy, The Observatories, Madingley Road, Cambridge, CB3 0HA, UK
s Pestalozzi- Gymnasium, 11, D-81247, München, Germany
t School of Biomedical Sciences, Perth, Curtin University, WA, Australia
u College of Physical and Mathematical Sciences, Australian National University, Canberra, Australia
v Henan Collaborative Innovation Center of Modern Biological Breeding, Henan Institute of Science and Technology, Xinxiang, 453003, China
w Department of Biochemistry, University of Alberta, Edmonton, AB T6G 2H7, Canada

Published in: Progress in Biophysics and Molecular Biology Volume 136, August 2018, Pages 3-23

Abstract

We review the salient evidence consistent with or predicted by the Hoyle-Wickramasinghe (H-W) thesis of Cometary (Cosmic) Biology. Much of this physical and biological evidence is multifactorial. One particular focus are the recent studies which date the emergence of the complex retroviruses of vertebrate

lines at or just before the Cambrian Explosion of ~500 Ma. Such viruses are known to be plausibly associated with major evolutionary genomic processes. We believe this coincidence is not fortuitous but is consistent with a key prediction of H-W theory whereby major extinction-diversification evolutionary boundaries coincide with virus-bearing cometary-bolide bombardment events. A second focus is the remarkable evolution of intelligent complexity (Cephalopods) culminating in the emergence of the Octopus. A third focus concerns the micro-organism fossil evidence contained within meteorites as well as the detection in the upper atmosphere of apparent incoming life-bearing particles from space. In our view the totality of the multifactorial data and critical analyses assembled by Fred Hoyle, Chandra Wickramasinghe and their many colleagues since the 1960s leads to a very plausible conclusion - life

* Corresponding author. CY O'Connor ERADE Village Foundation, Piara Waters,
WA, Australia.
E-mail address: ejsteele@cyo.edu.au (E.J. Steele).

Full article available from:
https://www.sciencedirect.com/science/article/pii/S0079610718300798

IN THE PRESS

THE WEEKEND AUSTRALIAN, APRIL 14-15, 2018
theaustralian.com.au

THE NATION 3

When I was contacted by Graham Lloyd we talked at length about "protective matrices" (all space derived organisms are associated with protective matrices - they have to be when you think about it). In the case of fertilised eggs of higher organisms ideal matrices are the cryo–megameteorites, effectively space "icebergs", which would be the ejecta from bolide collisions with some other (surface frozen) ocean–bearing moon, planet or comet carrying populations of fertilised eggs or embryos (possibly in their thousands and millions) which would be largely protected on impact in the new cosmic ocean-bearing habit, like Earth. None of this appeared in that news story. See attached and the scan of parts of page 1, 2 3 from *The Weekend Australian*. Note on page 1 of last Weekend's Australian is the UWA advert to flog their course to graduate and postgraduates- highlighting the research of a certain "Professor Roger Hart" who specialises in IVF. The extraordinary main finding of his research is that

Octopuses are from space, say scientists

EXCLUSIVE

GRAHAM LLOYD
ENVIRONMENT EDITOR

The evolution of life on Earth was spurred on by the bombardment from space of comets carrying viral genes and frozen eggs of complete species such as the octopus, a new multi-author paper has claimed.

Published in *Progress in Biophysics and Molecular Biology*, the paper looks at decades of research into cosmic biology.

It coincides with another peer-reviewed article by Russian scientists that found cosmic dust taken in swabs from the outside of the international space station contained DNA sequences typical of many terrestrial and ocean bacteria on Earth. The race is on to find out how it got there and was able to survive.

Lead authored by Australian molecular immunologist and evolutionist Edward J Steele, the international paper, Cause of the Cambrian Explosion — Terrestrial or Cosmic?, brings the pioneering work of Hoyle and Wickramasinghe on cosmic evolution firmly into the biomedical literature.

frozen and thawed embryos are far superior to fresh unfrozen embryos in human IVF. This makes sense in the cosmic paradigm. This is obviously important in embryo transfer in cattle I would think. *(Ted Steele)*

The Cambrian explosion is considered the most important evolutionary event in the history of life on Earth. Biology's "big bang", it happened 541 million years ago and is when most of the major groups of animals appear suddenly in the fossil record.

Professor Steele's findings challenge the conventional view that evolution of life on Earth was wholly terrestrial. The bottom line, says the new paper, is "current evidence suggests we came from space, we are made of viral genes, and eventually our evolutionary legacy would in full measure return to space".

The co-authors said: "In our considered opinion in confronting the wide range of scientific data, all the scientific and societal evidence seemingly points in one direction, an all-pervasive cosmic biology, mediated mainly by cometary transfers, being a driver for life on Earth. We believe the signs of this change are now so apparent that one of the biggest backflips in the history of science is now on our doorstep."

The paper's findings are so controversial some reviewers refused to consider it and called for publication to be withheld, journal editor Denis Noble said.

But he said when journals received way-out, speculative articles, they carried a heavy responsibility. "The first is to judge whether the theories proposed are empirical and testable," he said, suggesting one day this would be possible.

He believed science was advanced by critical review of controversial theories. "There really is no agreed theory on how life arose on Earth. We simply don't know. All theories therefore are currently 'way-out'."

Two reviewers were not convinced. Keith Baverstock of the Department of Environmental and Biological Sciences University of Eastern Finland, said the authors had put forward much evidence that would support an extraterrestrial origin of life, but not definitive evidence — evidence that could not be explained in any other terms.

Karin Moelling of the Max Planck Institute Berlin and Institute of Medical Microbiology, Zurich, said the article was worth thinking about, "yet the main statement about viruses, microbes and even animals coming to us from space, cannot be taken seriously," she said.

O'Connor family ingenuity shining still

By **MAL GILL**

PROBLEM-solving abilities inherited from legendary civil engineer Charles Yelverton O'Connor, along with genetics, are playing a role in agricultural research at North Dandalup.

"The Chief", as CY O'Connor was known during his tenure through the 1890s as WA's engineer in chief, overcame problems considered insurmountable by contemporaries while building Fremantle harbour and the Goldfields water supply scheme.

His great grandson, Roger Dawkins and his son John among others, are involved in a project trying to resolve potentially bigger problems – providing healthier, sustainable and more productive food sources using genetics to identify advantageous DNA differences.

North Dandalup is professor Dawkins' new base and he sees it developing as a scientific community involved in farming and agriculture-related research covering animal genetics, welfare and disease, perennial grasses, soil amendment, farm management systems and more as needs are identified.

Benefits will be for the Peel region initially, but potentially could be adapted for other food producing regions in Australia and around the world.

After a distinguished career in medical research and as an international authority on immunogenetics and autoimmune disease, professor Dawkins in retirement has turned his knowledge and experience to improving Peel region beef cattle, the meat they produce and the pastures they consume.

While recognised as a medical researcher and geneticist, he has a background and family history in agriculture.

"CY O'Connor was my mother's grandfather – her father was (Sir) Ernest Lee Steere, an innovative pastoralist and grazier," professor Dawkins said.

"On the other side, my father's side were agricultural people, one of them invented the first stump jump harrows, one was the first to produce Poll Dorset sheep.

"I've grown up listening to all these tales of invention so when I retired from The University of WA I took up agricultural research.

"My life has always had a rural background.

"We've always had farms and spent our holidays on farms or the mustering camp, with the family deeply involved in agriculture," he said.

Professor Dawkins is the visionary behind the establishment of the foreshadowed $26 million collaborative multidisciplinary CY O'Connor Centre for Innovation in Agriculture at North Dandalup.

The centre was founded last year by collaboration between Murdoch University, the CY O'Connor ERADE (Education, Research and Development, Employment) Village Foundation and the Dawkins' family company, Tillbrook Melaleuka Group (TMG).

The centre is constructing a laboratory beside a converted house used for offices and meetings at its initial five hectare site on Del Park Road.

Future growth plans involve the Peel Development Corporation (PDC) and Murray Shire.

A charitable foundation which mentors and nurtures scientists with capacity to take scientific discovery to commercial reality, the CY O'Connor ERADE Village Foundation's beginnings go back to 1983 as the Immunogenetics Research Foundation (IRF) which looked at responses to AIDS.

It now generates revenue from patents protecting its work.

Professor Dawkins is its founder, chairman and research director.

Deputy chairman is Paul Fitzpatrick, who was chairman of PDC until last September and deputy research director is Sally Lloyd, Murdoch University, who oversees research conducted by postgraduate students and sponsored by the foundation.

Nambeelup robotic dairy and beef cattle farmer Rob Giura is a board member.

Wednesday meetings at the CY O'Connor Centre for Innovation in

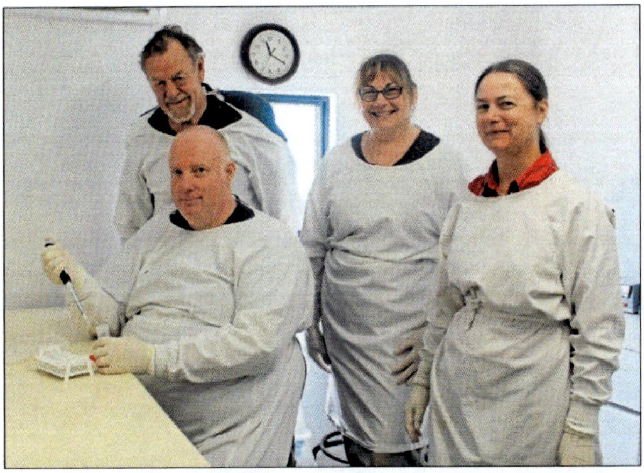

❐ Technician Matthew Nippierd (seated) prepares to extract short sections of DNA known as haplotypes to test the melting point of beef fat in an on-farm laboratory at Keysbrook. Watching are research director Roger Dawkins, technician Joanne Rollinson and deputy research director Sally Lloyd. A second laboratory funded by Murdoch University is being built nearby at the CY O'Connor Centre for Innovation in Agriculture.

Agriculture often attract local farmers interested in what regular guest speakers have to say.

Interaction with the community to learn from farmers' knowledge of local conditions and to share knowledge with them is part of Professor Dawkins' concept.

North Dandalup residents have already benefited from the relationship, with high speed broadband provided via a relocated tower funded as part of the research centre project.

Field trials are conducted on TMG farms on hill country at North Dandalup, on the Peel sand plain at nearby Nambeelup and at Waroona.

Professor Dawkins said farmers in the region have traditionally grazed cattle on the sand plain in summer, where they could find superficial water in swamp areas and moved them to hill blocks in winter to overcome a plains dietary minerals deficiency.

"We still do that," professor Dawkins said.

TMG runs herds of Japanese breeds Black Wagyu and Akaushi – sometimes called Red Wagyu – as well as Simmental cattle and son John oversees a vertically-integrated paddock-to-plate offshoot, with CY O'Connor Village Pub at Piara Waters and Hybla Tavern at Middleton Beach, Albany.

The tavern restaurants serve TMG's Melaleuka Melts long-fed marbled Black Wagyu and short-fed Simmental first cross Akaushi beef.

Grass-fed, marbled Akaushi beef is coming and TMG beef output has grown sufficiently so that a third tavern outlet is proposed.

The Melaleuka herds provide DNA for some of the research and DNA is collected from other herds.

Dr Lloyd said DNA samples from the Melaleuka herds go back 15 years, an invaluable archive few other research institutions have.

Scientific research is conducted in a converted dairy laboratory on the Nambeelup farm.

It will be supplemented by the new laboratory being built at the Del Park Road site.

Current projects include looking at the melting point of intramuscular fat in beef – Wagyu characteristics include marbling, which improves flavour and texture, and both Wagyu and Akaushi have fat which melts at below human body temperature.

This is important for health reasons, professor Dawkins said.

"We just need to get the genes from the Japanese cattle into the local cattle with sufficient certainty to be able to improve the quality of local beef," he said.

"If it (beef fat) melts at below human body temperature it can be readily metabolised and used.

"If, however, it is solid at that temperature, then it goes onto the vessels and creates stroke, heart disease and other problems.

"There is no question, the target is not only to produce more food, but healthier food.

"That's how we see it and that's why we are producing animals targeted at good health.

"We're already quite parochial in that we want to do the work here and have people trained here, farmers as savvy as they can be, but ultimately what we do has to translate to a wider area.

"We're local in focus but international in effect and the critical thing there is tracing.

"We know there is vastly more Australian Wagyu marketed in China than what is actually produced here.

"All sorts of meat is relabelled as Australian Wagyu.

"Our particular solution to that problem is to trace the DNA all the way down the chain."

A project the research centre is running is developing a simple, low-cost DNA trace, a sort of animal "fingerprint", professor Dawkins explained, which could potentially trace it from new-born calf through its life, through an abattoir and processing plant and onto a restaurant plate or supermarket shelf.

Apart from protecting country-of-origin and brand reputations in export markets where product substitution is rife, the trace could have benefits closer to home, he said.

"We've had experience at the CY O'Connor pub where at the abattoir the body has been switched," he said.

"Somebody has complained their steak is tough so we've taken a sample and it's not our steak.

"This is important to know because if it had been our steak that was tough, it could mean our breeding program has gone off the rails."

Researchers at the centre are also looking to identify genetic strains of Kikuyu that are able to adapt by sending roots down almost two metres to cope with the relatively rapid Peel sand plain water table movement across a range of about 1.5 metres from winter to summer.

If adaptable strains can be identified genetically and successfully bred it could produce more robust pastures which are less reliant on irrigation and better able to filter nutrients out of the water table before they reach the Peel Inlet and Harvey Estuary, Professor Dawkins said.

"This is a twin benefit we think," he said.

"The variety that has survived here from 40 years ago is the one which has put its roots down.

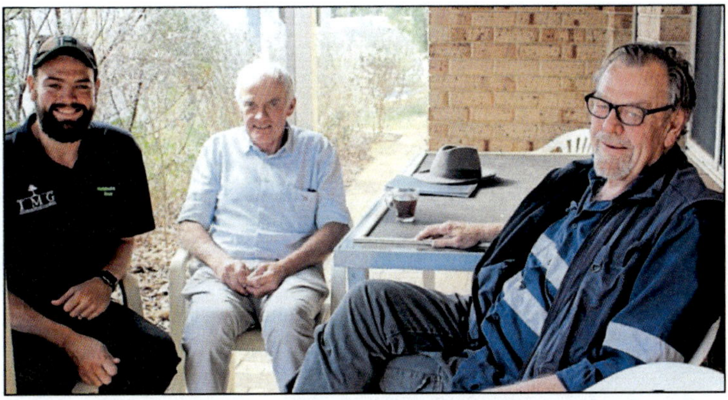

❒ John Dawkins (left), who runs a vertically-integrated paddock-to-plate family enterprise supplying beef to two tavern restaurants, his uncle Patrick Dawkins, who was involved in introducing Simmental cattle to WA and his father Roger Dawkins, who directs research at the CY O'Connor Centre for Innovation in Agriculture at North Dandalup.

"Then you find successful Kikuyu changes the soil ecology and now other grasses can grow here, you see perennial clovers and perennial Kikuyu which really puts a much more optimistic approach to agriculture in the region."

Professor Dawkins' concept of an agriculture research hub, complete with adjacent "incubator" village to accommodate researchers, located on farmland to facilitate trials and real-world applications of the science, has already been tested on the outskirts of Perth.

The CY O'Connor ERADE Village, including the pub and research facilities, was established on another Dawkins family farm 20 years ago at what is now suburban Piara Waters.

Urban encroachment at Piara Waters instigated the move to North Dandalup.

An accommodation village is also planned as part of the CY O'Connor Centre for Innovation in Agriculture.

It will be developed on a section of the Del Park Road site behind the new laboratory.

Professor Dawkins said there was also opportunity to rent or buy existing houses in North Dandalup to accommodate researchers and laboratory staff.

While a stand-alone project, the CY O'Connor Centre for Innovation in Agriculture is within the expanded 28,000ha Peel Food Zone proposed for intensive food production and related enterprises.

The food zone development, led by the Department of Primary Industries and Regional Development is a critical piece of PDC's $49.3m Transform Peel project.

As previously reported in *Farm Weekly*, Transform Peel is proposed to culminate in 2050 with estimated economic output of $1.2 billion a year and creation of 33,000 new jobs through diversifying the region's economy, protecting its environment and encouraging and enabling investment in innovative technology and food production systems.

Part of the Transform Peel project is a proposed 1000ha business park with a focus on food manufacturing and processing, logistics and supporting commercial and light industrial activities to be developed by LandCorp on the western edge of the food zone.

In conjunction with the Singapore Centre for Research Innovation Productivity and Technology, PDC has completed a feasibility study into smart urban farm factories.

It is a partner in the North Dandalup research centre as part of its Transform Peel commitment to encouraging innovation and science in the region.

WHILE technology is touted as the future in agriculture, it will be scientific researchers solving problems that determines agriculture's future, according to Roger Dawkins.

As founder, chairman and research director of the CY O'Connor ERADE Village Foundation, professor Dawkins wants to ensure university students and post graduate students are aware of the potential for scientific problem solvers, particularly in agriculture, to find a rewarding career.

"We need to get across the message to younger people wanting to get trained in the newer aspects of farming that we (foundation) have scholarships and traineeships, but we don't have any applicants," he said.

"Why is that?

"Perhaps it's because we haven't told anyone.

"We advertise (on foundation literature), but you have to already know us before you see that.

"We know from our practical experience there are plenty of bright kids who could be engaged, they love cattle, they love sheep, there's a potential pool of people that for some reason they're not engaged in farming at the present.

"We've got to work out a way of getting them involved and maintaining sufficient interest to see some sort of career.

"We want it to be problem solving," he said.

The CY O'Connor ERADE Village Foundation annually offers up to five $30,000 innovation awards to inventors with research and development projects.

Applications should include a description of the solution to any problems in fields such as biomedicine, agriculture, environmental science and sustainable energy, that the inventors are working on.

The awards package includes a 12-month licence to use the ERADE village facilities, including a live-in research studio, access to staff supervision and shared facilities including laboratories, computing, technical assistance and intellectual property management.

Independently of the CY O'Connor ERADE Village Foundation, the AL & M Dawkins Foundation sponsors WA biomedical research for up to $200,000 each year.

❒ For information: contact the CY O'Connor ERADE Village Foundation on 9397 1556 or visit cyovillage.com.au.

Farm Weekly article, May 3 2018

SW clear of cattle disease

David Charlesworth

Things are looking positive for WA cattle producers with Statewide testing for Bovine Johne's Disease 76 per cent complete and so far negative.

Department of Primary Industries and Regional Development Animal Disease Control manager Bruce Twentyman said 100 properties in WA had undergone voluntary testing of Johne's Disease, 10 of which were beef and dairy herds in the Harvey-Waroona region.

Dr Twentyman said Johne's disease was an incurable bacterial infection which caused chronic weight loss and took a number of years to build in a cow's system.

"In the short term it really impacts on production and the health and welfare of the animal," he said.

Dr Twentyman said 76 per cent of the properties had been sampled, with the program expected to finish before the end of the year.

"It's an industry-run scheme that the Government is managing for industry," Dr Twentyman said.

"There have been no positive tests of Johne's to date, that is looking very positive for WA."

Dr Twentyman said the testing was on behalf of the Cattle Industry Funding Scheme to inform future decisions made on biosecurity controls. "It's part of our surveillance to allow industry to make decisions about controlling Johne's disease in the State," he said.

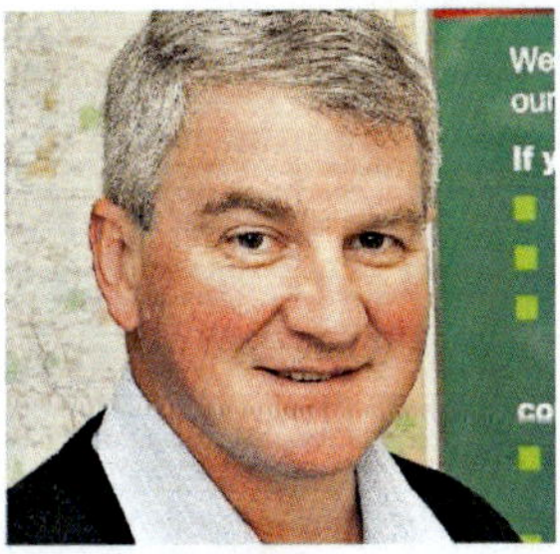

Bruce Twentyman

Biosecurity controls of Johne's Disease were deregulated in other States in 2016.

Dr Twentyman said WA producers had decided not to deregulate until they had more information on the actual prevalence of the disease in the State. "It will be an industry decision," he said.

Dr Twentyman said in order to institute border controls and restrictions, WA needed to demonstrate it had a negligible presence of the disease.

"We can't introduce border restrictions unless there's a very low level of Johne's in cattle, otherwise it's a restriction of trade," he said.

Dr Twentyman said new national arrangements for Johne's had categorised all forms of it together, so WA was no longer considered free of Johne's because of the ovine, or sheep, variant.

An additional 77 cattle properties had completed voluntary testing for a Johne's Beef Assurance Score and were also negative.

Producers were automatically given the highest score as long as their property did not have Ovine Johne's disease, present in sheep.

Testing which confirms no presence of Johne's enabled producers to maintain that top rating for the next three years.

"It will give producers a marketing advantage, especially if they are selling interstate or selling to other producers in WA," Dr Twentyman said.

This advice is welcome and raises the issue of whether WA should encourage vaccination as a means of protecting its naive and susceptible herd from the future unintentional introduction of the disease. CIA is in discussion with the authorities so as to weigh the pros and cons of a research project. A critical issue for exporters is whether it is possible to confirm the distinction between natural infection and positive serology induced by the vaccine.

R L Dawkins

Countryman edition, 14 June 2018, Page 29 ADDED IN PROOF

Featured Articles

Why is Dr Sally interested in EMUS, MACADEMIAS, OLIVES and WAGYU?

What do these have in common?

Low Melting Temperature and therefore healthy fat.

EMUS are the survivors of the Dinosaurs. Rather than being threatened with extinction they are everywhere and seem to be very adaptable to present day hazards. Just this week, I counted 20 at MUNDUP, 20 at POLLARDS and about the same at ROEBROOKS.

It is not as though we have decided to preserve them. To the contrary, they have made the decision to live with us. In fact, although Lindsay, John and Ben think of themselves as dedicated beef breeders, they are feeding more emus, kangaroos and feral pigs than cattle.

So, can we adapt to the reality that near urban farming is fraught with these invasive and successful pests plus even more successful feral humans and, as it is, flammable road verges which destroy fences every year.

EMUS are interesting. They convert pretty well everything they can find partly by eating stones which lodge in the gizzard and therefore facilitate the use of otherwise indigestible left-overs, like wood and insect husks, which cattle will not eat. More impressive, they deposit low TM fat which is used in hard times including the almost 2 months when the male incubates a dozen eggs. Often, because the males have not been on Facebook, they accept eggs of diverse parentage, perhaps explaining why EMUS retain a very high level of adaptability and survival.

Remarkably, essentially all the low TM fat is stored subcutaneously allowing release when required for survival. Wagyu, according to current thinking, have been selected to store their low Tm lipids in muscle so they can pull ploughs through rice paddies and serendipitously provide healthy and tasty steak.

The fact is that EMUs have beaten WAGYU in their capacity to desaturase fat Remarkably, according to popular media and marketing, 42% of the subcutaneous fat in EMUS is C18 oleic acid as found in olives and macadamia. Of course, the low Tm fat is in the wrong place if you are after a marbled steak.

May be this is why Dr Sally is interested.

But, if she is thinking of setting up an EMU farm, determining the parentages and defining the metabolic pathways plus the relevant haplotypes, she will need some really bright committed students and therefore some financial commitments, which I will match.

Professor Roger L. Dawkins

A 'blast from the past' and so, what now?

by Jerzy K. Kulski, BSc (Hons) & PhD
(retired with adjunct position at The University of Western Australia, School of Psychiatry and Clinical Neurosciences).

Regulation and Immunity

The HCP5 lncRNA gene is the non-coding remnant of an ancient viral sequence: A scientific memory from the nineties at the CMII, a precursor to the C. Y. O'Connor ERADE village.

References:

Kulski J. K., Gaudieri, S., Inoko, H., and Dawkins, R. L. (1999). Comparison between two HERV-rich regions within the major histocompatibility complex. Journal of Molecular Evolution, 48, 675-683.

Kulski J. K. and Dawkins, R. L. (1999). The P5 multicopy gene family in the MHC is related in sequence to human endogenous retroviruses HERV-L and HERV-16. Immunogenetics, 49, 404-412.

Professor Roger Dawkins requested a scientific memory from me to add to his annual report about our time together in the late 90s at the Centre of Molecular Instrumentation and Immunology (CMII), which was one of the precursors to the

C. Y. O'Connor ERADE village. I have provided the two references above as an example of a '*blast from the past*' and with an account below about what new information or developments resulted from our 1999 publication on the P5 multicopy gene family. This illustrates in part how slowly the wheels of scientific development can turn and progress with respect to following up on original research findings.

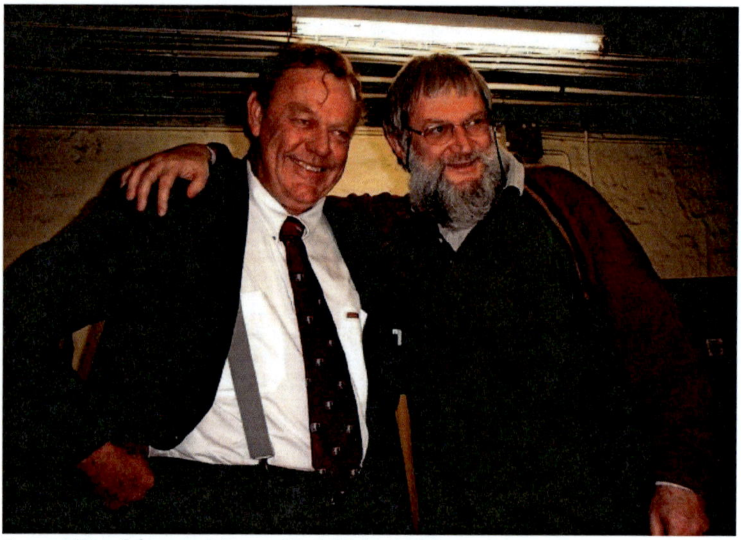

Roger Dawkins and Jerzy Kulski in 1999

When I was at CMII for three years, the studies I shared with Professor Dawkins and his group mostly involved the newly developed art and science of bioinformatics, that is, the analysis of the very first available human genomic sequences using computers as well as pencil and paper to work out the human Major Histocompatibility Complex (MHC, also known as the HLA) genomic structure, gene duplications and the role of ancient retroelements (fossilised viral RNA sequences) in driving the duplication, organisation and evolution of the innate and adaptive immunity and transplantation genes located on the short arm of chromosome six. We overturned a number of the traditional beliefs of that time including that it was not just single genes that were duplicated in the MHC genomic region. Instead, we showed that it was long extended regions of multiple, linked gene structures (haplotypes) located between and including fossilised retroelements that were duplicated and rearranged over millions of years of evolution within and between the different hominoid species.

During our five-years together, two at Royal Perth Hospital and then three at the CMII, Professor Dawkins and I co-authored at least 20 papers on the organization and generation of the gene structure of the HLA genomic region, many of them subsequently remembered and referenced in follow-up publications by other scientists constructing their own research edifices with some help from our initial contributions. One of our papers was unusual for its time because we found and reported that all the members of the family of the duplicated P5 genes in the HLA class I locus were actually repeat sequences of a modified ancient retroviral sequence known as ERVL/16. The Pontarotti group in France discovered the P5 gene family in 1993, and a year later they showed that one of these duplicated genes P5.1 was expressed as a long non-coding RNA in various human cells and tissues, whereas the other family members remained silent. During the course of our DNA sequence investigation of the HLA class I genomic region while looking for evidence of ancient retroviral insertions using a public database of known endogenous and exogenous viral sequences, we discovered that the P5 gene family of non-coding genes was in fact composed of the retroviral sequence ERVL/16 (Kulski J. K., Gaudieri, S., Inoko, H., and Dawkins, R. L. 1999, above). In our follow-up paper '*The P5 multicopy gene family in the MHC is related in sequence to human endogenous retroviruses HERV-L and HERV-16*' we confirmed that the P5.1 sequence has its roots in an ancient retrovirus that evolved over millions of years into variant (polymorphic) forms with new molecular functions, and we deduced that this sequence probably evolved in primates as an antiviral gene with a role in immunity to retrovirus infections.

The last time that Professor Dawkins and I discussed the P5.1 sequence was with Pierre Pontarotti, the French discoverer of the duplicated P5 gene family, at an enjoyable CMII retreat in Albany in 1999. Since then, the P5.1 DNA sequence has had an official name change and it is now known as HCP5, and it is classified as a long non-coding RNA (lncRNA). That is, it is a genomic sequence transcribed like a gene, but the generated transcript (lncRNA) is not translated into a functional protein (the 'gene' product is RNA and not a protein). In 1999, apart from HCP5, few other lncRNA had been previously described. HCP5 is therefore one of the few earliest examples of a lncRNA sequence with unknown function. However, soon after the new millennium, with the sudden development of next generation sequencing methods, there was an enormous discovery explosion of tens of thousands of different lncRNA sequences in various mammalian species. We now know that the lncRNA sequences are the most numerous and functionally diverse class of RNAs, and they are as rich, numerous and functionally versatile as the proteome. Moreover, they are key regulators of gene expression at multiple levels of cellular genetic activity and control.

Recent studies have confirmed that the HCP5 lncRNA sequence indeed does affect the HIV viral load in infected individuals as we first indicated in our 1999 paper, although the actual mechanism of action remains unknown. Others have shown that variants of the HCP5 sequence are strongly associated with HIV disease progression, HIV anti-viral abacavir and nevirapine drug sensitivity, psoriasis, susceptibility to herpes zoster virus and various types of cancers. A few years ago, in 2016, the Chinese group of Yunhui Liu demonstrated that the HCP5 transcribed sequence interacted with a microRNA sequence and the Runt-related transcriptional regulator RUNX1 in a feedback loop to regulate the malignant behavior of glioma cells of the brain. Moreover, an earlier 2014 study at the NIH in the USA showed that RUNX1 binds to HIV LTR sequences to suppress transcription and regulate CD4+ T cell function. Thus, HCP5 looks like it could be a potential regulator of HIV infections and T-cells and cancers by acting via the RUNX1 and microRNA transcriptional regulators in a process of feedback loops. On this basis, HCP5 might even be developed as an attenuated viral sequence to treat cancer or help in the clearance of HIV-I to treat AIDS.

Although Professor Dawkins and I were not able to follow up on our 1999 publication to better demonstrate the importance of the P5.1 (HCP5) sequence in human health, we and the Pontarotti group have led the way for others to continue on with the work and to recognise and acknowledge our papers as providing important contributions towards the better understanding of the structure and molecular role of the HCP5 DNA sequence. However, some researchers refer to our unique findings in their publications without ever citing our papers. For example, Crosslin *et al* (2015, Genes and Immunity 16: 1-7) write about HCP5 in their paper on the genetic variation in the HLA region associated with susceptibility to herpes zoster without referencing us, and yet they provide us with the following statement to read as a matter of fact: '*Given the fact that HCP5 is non-coding and is related to human endogenous retroviruses, we hypothesize that this region could be serving a host-driven regulatory function for herpes zoster.*' In this regard, even though our paper was not referenced, the rephrasing of the Google Scholar meme to '*stand on the shoulders of past researchers*' still rings true for our 1999 papers and those of others like the Pontarotti group who previously worked on the unusual origin and function of the HCP5 DNA structure. We now look forward to finding out from those very busy bees at the C. Y. O'Connor ERADE village what lncRNAs and if anything, similar to the HCP5 lncRNA sequence might exist in the genomic and transcriptional regulation of muscle marbling, lipid metabolism and Wagyu beef growth. Unfolding the research findings from the past often connects them in some unexpected and wonderful ways to as yet unsolved scientific questions. In this case, the answers will likely depend on the Centre for Innovative Agriculture finding and providing stable financial support for students and researchers interested in asking and answering the challenging scientific questions required to open up new developments in Western Australian agricultural and cattle industry, business, education and research.

To quote the Nobel Prize recipient Albert Szent-Gyorgi, '*Research is to see what everybody else has seen, and to think what nobody else has thought.*' The findings of our research in the late 1990s are now published, set in stone, old fashioned and for everybody else to see and consider in wonderment or as simple cold facts. While it can be fun and informative to dwell on old memories and achievements, Professor Dawkins and the C. Y. O'Connor ERADE village have new and important ideas and outcomes to pursue and to accomplish through sound financial support, reason, innovation, change and value adding by the compounding law of multiple progression.

Travel Reports

Australian Wagyu Conference and Tour 2017

Sally Lloyd

28th April -1st May
Goorambat Wagyu and Cutting Edge Genomics
Laboratory Inspection, Equipment Set up
Training of staff in DNA and Fat extraction, Melting point measurement, PCR and C19 marker analysis.
30th April: Presentation of CYO Research projects (Haplotype approach, Chr 19 haplotypes for muscle and fat DNA markers for scur location on Chromosome 19, Tm comparison of breeds, to Healthy Beef Collaboration. (Dom Bayard, Keith Hammond, Sarah Hammond,).

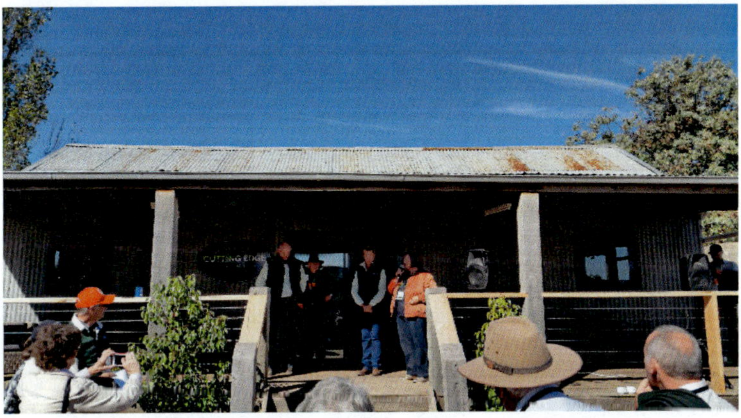

Dom and Jo Bayard address the crowds in front of their new on-farm laboratory

Adopting Smart Beef Cattle Feeding Techniques,

Sally Lloyd

1 to 5, June, Seminar and Training Program - Adopting Smart Beef Cattle Feeding Techniques Suranaree University of Technology, Nakhon Ratchasima, Thailand sponsored by the Food and Fertiliser Technology Center for the Asian and Pacific Region.

Researchers and industry representatives from Thailand, Japan, Korea, Taiwan, Philippines, Vietnam, Malaysia and Indonesia presented reports on state of the beef industries in their respective countries, and research into feeding techniques. Feeding techniques included various types of

fermented mixed rations which made use of local food production waste streams.
Reducing methane emissions and improving feed efficiency was another area of focus with various
The Suranee university and near-by Khon Khaen university were experimenting with crossbreeding local cattle to native cattle breeds and Brahman crossbreeds. Visitors from Japan were involved in research collaborations but could not supply Japanese genetic material. Most frozen semen used for the cross breeding came from Australian Wagyu Bulls.

2 June :Seminar series to expert group
3 June :presentations to 200 participants to include regional farmers, extension workers, and animal feeding experts from universities and NRS in the AP region.
After the conference I travelled to Khon Khaen University to visit the resesarch group of Chanvit Leewat. I presented to the group "Haplotypes for Type, Degree and Rate of Marbling in Cattle are Syntenic with Human Muscular Dystrophy". I also made contact with Dr. Kritapon Sommart, of the animal production group at Khon Khaen, and toured their facilities.

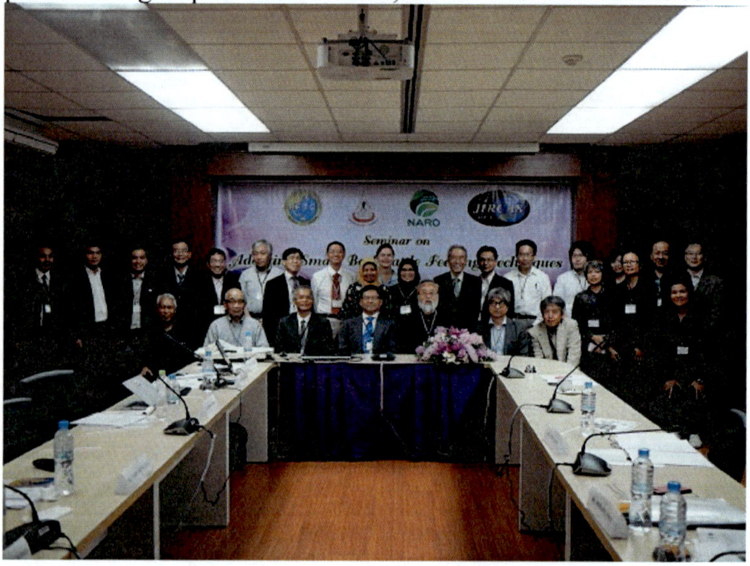

Japan Wagyu Tour

John Dawkins – TMG, Primary Industry Partner

In September last year, I had the opportunity to go with the Australian Wagyu Association on a tour of Japan to gain a greater understanding of the breeding, feeding, processing and retailing of Japanese Wagyu beef with the tour concluding at the Zenkyo (5-yearly Wagyu "Olympics").

Breeding

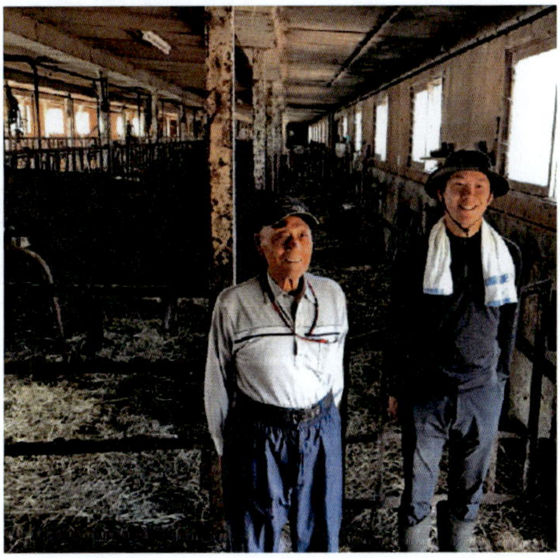
Takeda-san and his grandson

We visited almost a dozen prefectures and many black wagyu producers with the highlight being Takeda-san and his grandson in Shiraoi. Takeda-san believes in crossing a number of wagyu bloodlines in order to maintain a balance of desirable traits and follows a strict rotation (known as the Takeda rotation) rather than the more traditional idea of sticking to your prefecture's line (or introducing Tajima only). Takeda-san played a role in getting wagyu cattle out to Australia (including those which led to Itoshigenami Jnr) and is always helpful to Aussie's. He believes that his cattle are marbled by 20 months with the final 12 months for increasing carcass size.

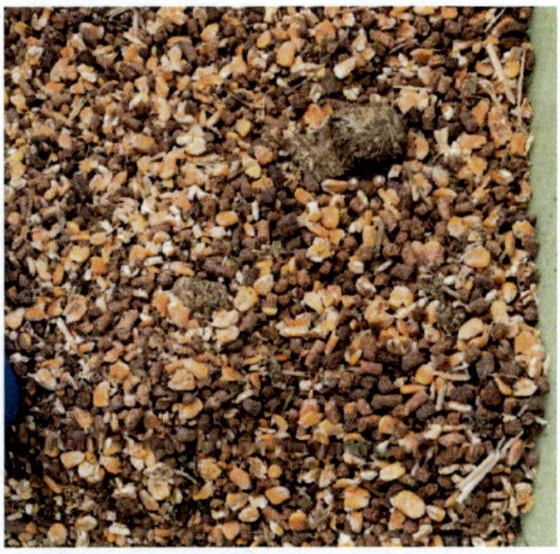
Japanese Feed Ration

Feeding

For the most part, the breeders/producers were feeding their own cattle but we did see a number of dedicated feedlots. Larger facilities, as we can find at home, are rare but do exist and include one we visited which was importing Australian wagyu cattle. Interestingly, as they were spending the majority of their lives in Japan prior to slaughter, they are able to marketed as Japanese wagyu beef (despite Australia not having wagyu cattle to their mind). Most feeding operations use 3 rations being for (roughly) the first year of life, the second year of life and then through to slaughter (30-36 months). The rations follow the general rule of higher protein early and higher energy late and include corn.

Processing

We had the opportunity to visit two meat processing facilities, one in the capital and one in a rural area. For the most part, the producers/feeders maintain ownership of the cattle through the slaughter process and up until wholesalers purchase by anonymous auction. Soon after slaughter, a Japanese Meat Grading Association employee grades the animal and the lineage and carcass data are released to the wholesalers. At approximately 2 weeks on the hook, the sale occurs and prices of up to $20,000 AUD equivalent per body are common. Being a grader is a true profession and apparently requires something similar to a undergraduate university degree to enable registration. We also were able to witness (at the rural facility) the per-body boning into the Japanese cut-up. It was labour intensive but allows the body to be used to its full potential.

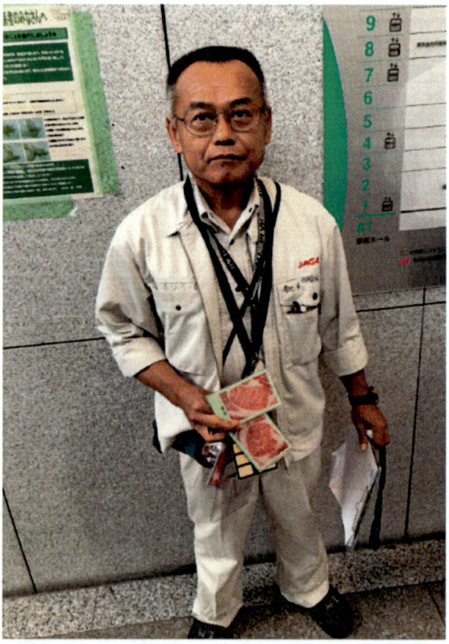

Japanese Meat Grading Association employee with reference cards for marbling

Retail

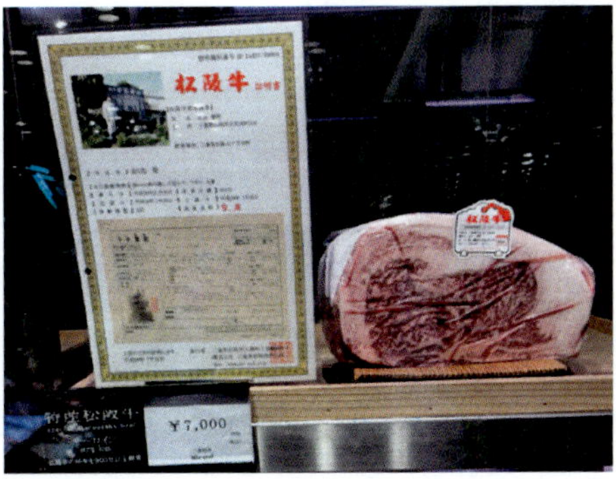

Wagyu meat retailing at $800/kg

The most striking aspect of the retail (aside from the obvious extreme prices) was the willingness to pay for 'lesser' cuts. While some steak cuts could go for as much as over $800/kg generally the A5 sweet cuts would be ~$200/kg at the prime retailers. By comparison, even rissole type products could go for as much as $100/kg! The packaging and presentation of the beef was also very impressive. It did turn out, however, that A5 wagyu beef is something that the general local would almost never experience.

Zenkyo

The Zenkyo is held every 5 years and has a number of components:

- Live cattle judging
- Carcass competition judging
- Trade show / promotional stalls
- Presentations
- Sale

It was exciting to see that a number of the issues we are investigating were front of mind at the Zenkyo such as melting temp of fat (see right - % oleic acid on the x axis), flavour/taste/VFA's and traceability through the supply chain.

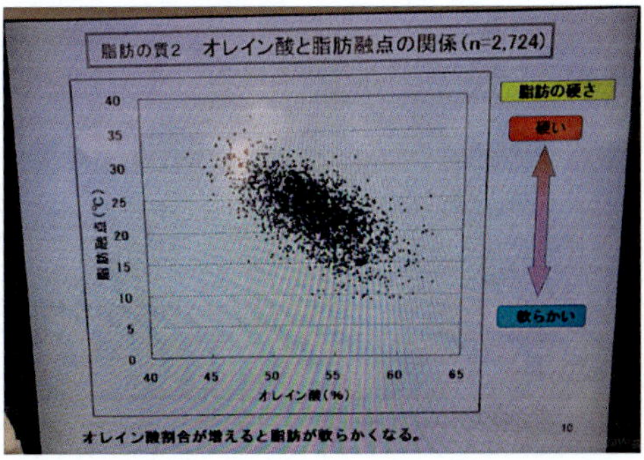

Presentation at Zenkyo showing the relationship between melting temperature of fat (vertical axis) and % oleic acid (horizontal axis)

Events

CYO' Connor Foundation - Murdoch University, Centre for Innovation in Agriculture launch, 13th April 2017

On the 13th of April 2017 a signing ceremony took place at CY O'Connor Tavern, launching the Centre for Innovation in Agriculture. Murdoch University and CY O'Connor Foundation signed an agreement, of which will ensure a Centre for Innovation many years to come.

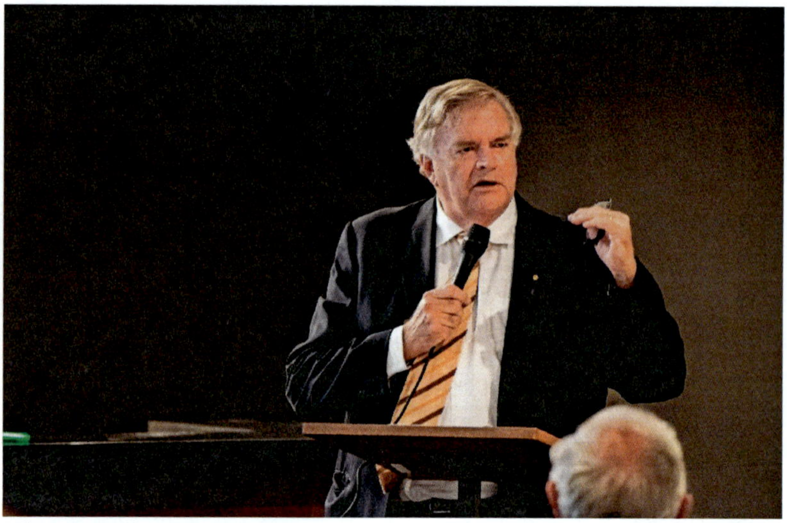

His Excellency The Honourable Kim Beazley, AC, the Governor General of Western Austrlia, Speaks at the CIA Launch.

Murdoch
UNIVERSITY

MEMORANDUM OF UNDERSTANDING

Between

Murdoch University of 90 South Street, Murdoch, Western Australia ABN 61 616 369 313 («Murdoch »)

and

The C Y O'Connor ERADE Village Foundation of Level 2, 100 Havelock St, Weste Perth, Western Australia ABN 67 161 830 965

And

T M Group WA Pty Ltd of PO Box 5100, Canningvale 6155, Western Australia ABN 18 605 884 302

1. **INTRODUCTION**

1.1. Murdoch University, C Y O'Connor ERADE Village Foundation and T M Group (hereafter 'the Parties') have a common purpose in the development and dissemination of knowledge and in supporting and undertaking research and training relevant to the communities ithey operate in.

1.2. The Parties have decided that they will enter into this Memorandum of Understanding (hereafter 'Memorandum') for cooperation in achieving their objectives. They have entered into this Memorandum to create an institute from which such collaboration may be developed and to facilitate the establishment of a contractual relationship between them leading to the conduct of one or more collaborative activities.

2. **DEFINITIONS**

2.1. **Agreement** means an legally abiding agreement entered into the by the Parties which governs a Project which may or may not include a third party.

2.2. **Background Intellectual Property** means any intellectual property already owned by or licensed to a Party prior to the signing of this Memorandum, or created or acquired by a Party independent of the Memorandum.

2.3. **Developed Intellectual Property** means intellectual property that is discovered, developed or has otherwise come into existence as a result of, for the purpose of, or in connection with the performance of a project, and excludes background intellectual property.

2.4. **Intellectual Property** includes all present and future rights, title and interests in and to inventions, knowhow, patents, trade marks, designs, copyright, domain names, and business names (and includes the right to apply for registration of such rights). It does not include confidential information or non-assignable rights such as moral rights.

2.5. **Party** means a party to this Memorandum and Parties means all of them.

2.6. **Project** means individual projects agreed to by the parties from time to.

2.7. **Student** means any Higher Degree by Research student.

3. **NATURE OF COLLABORATION**

3.1. The parties will discuss opportunities for collaboration in the area of primary food production, including sustainable farming, biosecurity and livestock production, in the Peel region. Such opportunities will include:

3.1.1. An annual contribution of $1 million as approved by all the parties, not including GST, from the C Y O'Connor ERADE Village Foundation to Murdoch University towards the costs of the collaboration renewable for 5 years. Murdoch University indirect costs or overheads will not be applied to this contribution. Specifically staff costs will be limited to salary and superannuation.

Page: 2

3.1.2. The naming of a research entity of Murdoch University at a location at the North Dandalup town site, on land provided by the C Y O'Connor ERADE Village Foundation or TMG to Murdoch University. Subject to appropriate subdivision, an area may be donated to Murdoch University.

3.1.3. Appointment of C Y O'Connor ERADE Village Foundation staff and members at Murdoch University to facilitate research and the supervision of Higher Degree by Research students, in accordance with relevant Murdoch University policy and procedures and supervision guidelines.

3.1.4. Appointment of Murdoch University staff in honorary positions to C Y O'Connor ERADE Village Foundation.

3.1.5. Research training through Higher Degree by Research scholarships, to be supervised by C Y O'Connor ERADE Village Foundation staff and members holding appointments with Murdoch University and Murdoch University staff holding appointments as Fellows of C Y O'Connor ERADE Village Foundation.

3.1.6. Joint research activity, including grant funding applications, research translation and Developed Intellectual Property.

3.1.7. Access to facilities and support services at Murdoch campuses, including research ethics processes.

3.1.8. Use of the T M Group WA Pty Ltd farms and research and training facilities on terms to be agreed on a project by project basis.

3.1.9. Establishment of a Board to govern activity and facilitate stakeholder engagement within the Peel Region, and beyond. The Board will be comprise equal number of representatives from each party.

3.1.10. Contribution of block grant funding from Murdoch University derived from the Parties joint activity, to support the aims of the collaboration

The parties will jointly appoint a steering committee to oversee implementation of this Memorandum of Understanding, and to consider the areas of research to be the subject of the collaboration. The steering committee will be made up four nominees from each of Murdoch University and C Y O'Connor ERADE Village Foundation. In the absence of any member, deputies may be appointed. Prof Morrison shall be one of Murdoch University's nominees and shall chair the Committee.

As a means of expediting the implementation of the Collaboration, Murdoch University will appoint existing staff of C Y O'Connor ERADE Village Foundation as staff members of Murdoch University on the Foundation's undertaking to meet salary and superannuation costs. Murdoch University will appoint an additional three mutually agreed support staff to service the requirements of the collaboration either from existing supernumerary Murdoch staff, by secondment or external appointment as the case may be. The salary and superannuation costs may be taken from the Foundation's contribution if required.

3.4. Where an activity may give rise to rights and obligations between the parties, a legally binding agreement shall be negotiated and entered into.

4. CONFIDENTIALITY

4.1. Each party shall only use the other party's confidential information, which is communicated to it in connection with this Memorandum for the purpose for which it was communicated or with the permission of the communicating party.

5. INTELLECTUAL PROPERTY

5.1. Nothing in this Memorandum alters or affects the ownership of any intellectual property, which is communicated by one party to another.

5.2. Nothing in this Memorandum affects the ownership of any Background Intellectual Property.

5.3. The Parties agree that the rights to Developed Intellectual Property will be negotiated and set out in any Agreement entered into by the Parties. The intent by the Parties, subject to 5.2 and 6., is to assign any Developed Intellectual Property to the C Y O'Connor ERADE Village Foundation arising from activities governed by an Agreement, with royalty licensing terms to be negotiated and agreed.

5.4. To the extent necessary to comply with any Agreement entered into by the Parties, Murdoch University will agree to arrange for any Student involved in a Project to assign all associated Developed Intellectual Property (other than copyright in a thesis) to Murdoch University so as to be dealt with as specified under this Memorandum..

6. GRANT FUNDING

The Parties acknowledge that Murdoch University may apply for Grant Funding to support activities, in collaboration or not with the Partiės or third parties. If that application is made and is successful then the Parties will amend or replace any relevant Agreement on the basis that the amended or replacement Agreement will be broadly consistent and will include changes to ensure compliance and consistency with any Grant Funding Agreement, such as:

6.1.1. a requirement of all Parties to comply with the Grant Funding Agreement;

6.1.2. the inclusion of clauses to allow for the management of Grant funds in accordance with the requirements of the Grant Funding Agreement;

6.1.3. allowing for reporting to the Commonwealth and subsequent use of reports by the Commonwealth;

6.1.4. the inclusion of any indemnities, assurances and notification requirements consistent with or required by the Grant Funding Agreement;

Page: 4

6.1.5. a requirement to comply with the Grant Funder open access policy in respect of publications arising from the Project;

6.1.6. a requirement to give credit to the Grant Funder in any publication arising from the Project;

6.1.7. joining any additional collaborators as Parties; and

6.1.8. an acknowledgement that nothing will prevent the lodgment of data, specimens or samples collected during, or resulting from, the Project with an appropriate museum or archive in Australia in accordance with arrangements made between the Investigators and the Grant Funder.

7. **OTHER ACTIVITY**

7.1. Each party will assign a person to be in charge of the implementation and maintenance of this Memorandum and to negotiate and manage any changes to this Memorandum.

7.2. Both parties will consider the development of joint proposals for the conduct of research, knowledge transfer, service or entrepreneurial activities.

7.3. Both parties will endeavor to include the other party's web-page as a hypertext link (or hot link) from their home page or from related sub-pages

8. **MISCELLANEOUS**

8.1. This Memorandum will be effective for five years as from the date of signing.

8.2. The renewal of this Memorandum shall be reviewed by the two parties in writing no less than six months prior to the natural termination of the current Agreement.

8.3. Either party may terminate this Memorandum by giving written notice to the other party 6 months prior to the termination.

8.4. This Memorandum does not constitute any financial commitment by either party.

8.5. This Memorandum is not intended to be legally binding and nothing in it shall be taken to create any legally binding contract, agreement or relationship between the parties.

8.6. Upon signature of this Memorandum, the parties agree to a joint public announcement.

9. **EXECUTION**

9.1. Executed as a memorandum of understanding by the parties:

Executed for and on behalf of **Murdoch University** by:

Professor Chris Hutchison

Name (print) Signature

Director Research & Innovation 9/3/2017

Position Title (print) Dated

Executed for and on behalf of **C Y O'Connor ERADE Village Foundation** by:

ANTHONY JAMES LLOYD

Name (print) Signature

VICE CHAIRMAN 9/3/2017

Position Title (print) Dated

Executed for and on behalf of **T M Group WA Pty Ltd** by:

Roger. L. Dawkins

Name (print) Signature

Director 9/3/17

Position Title (print) Dated

Page: 6

Weekly Research Meetings

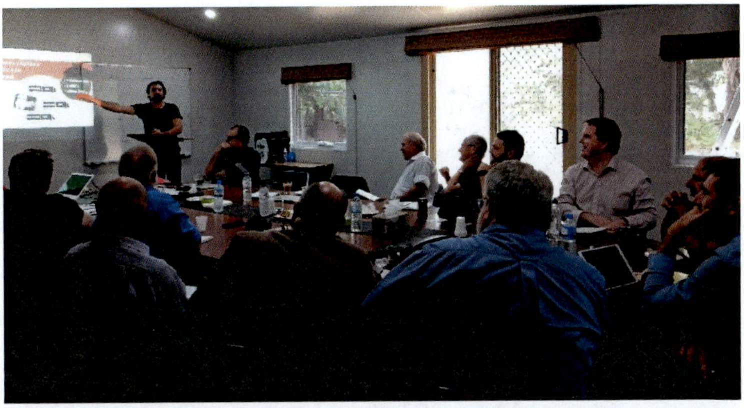

Each Wednesday throughout the year, CY O'Connor Foundation holds a 1 hour research meeting to share knowledge and research opportunities. This year the location of meetings was established in the new Centre for Innovation in Agriculture, North Dandalup.

Topics discussed throughout 2017 have included:
Beef feeding trials
Ethics requirements
Metabolomics in Beef Marbling
Bovine Johne's Disease
Business Incubators
Potential of solar and battery power in Farming systems
Camel Dairy farming opportunities in the South West
Tracing provenance in Foods
Transform Peel project
Local employment opportunities

> *Attending the Wednesday research meetings at North Dandalup provided my team with important opportunities to share the results of our investigations into the Peel Food Zone with local farmers. We listened to locals with many combined years of experience farming in the Peel and their feedback has influenced future planning for the Peel Food Zone.*

Heather Percy
Manager Peel Food Zone project

Professor Roger Dawkins visits North Dandalup Primary School

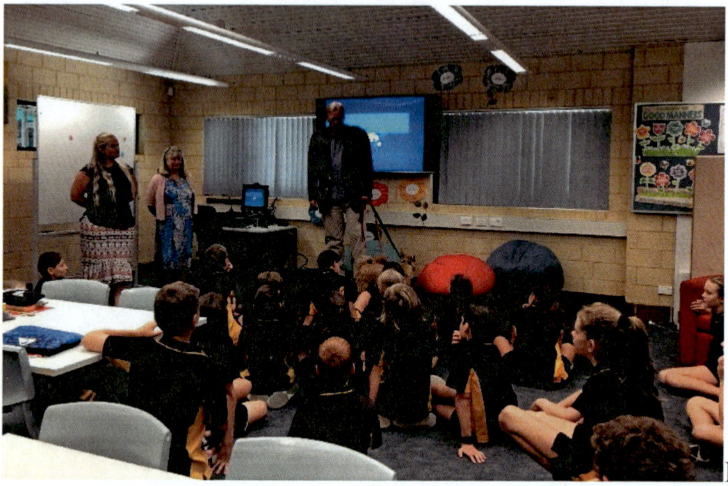

Professor Roger Dawkins visited North Dandalup Primary School in 2017

The students took a keen interest learning what is involved in a research Centre and working on a farm.

They also enjoyed the professor's dogs.

Scientific Retreats 2017

13th-15th July: Future Proofing

Rose Cottage, Melalueka Stud, North Dandalup

Symposium 1: Measuring Meat Quality

Wagyu genetics and healthy fats *Sally Lloyd*
The Akaushi breed: Origins, benefits and future *Aaron Cooper*
Measuring marbling and meat quality *Dave Pethick*
Methods of carcass and live animal Tm Measurement *Sally Lloyd*

Symposium 2: Ruminant Nutrition

Melaleuka Feed Trials – Observations *Lindsay Baker*
Melaleuka Feed Trials – Analysis *John Dawkins*
Melaleuka Feed Trials –Monitoring Retinol, Tm and Marbling *Jose Valenzuela*
Feeding the Rumen *Herbert Rebhan*

Symposium 3: Business Incubator Proposals

CYO Business Incubators – past and future *Roger Dawkins*
Available support for innovative businesses *Roban-Lynne Clarke*
North Dandalup Agriculture Research and Innovation Precinct *Tim Connolly*
Intellectual property for haplotype tracing, provenance and quality *Roger Dawkins*
Research abattoir for improved processing and labelling *Rob Giura*
In vivo testing of meat quality and safety *Herbert Rebhan*
Testing for BJD *Roger Dawkins*
R and D in building materials and servicing *Rob Giura*
Insect protein for safe feeding of livestock: avoidance of prions *Paula Pownall*
Salt water battery *Manickam Minakshi*
Adapting pasture mixes *Tony Lloyd*
Mycobacterial protein for prevention and treatment of BJD and Scurs *Dom Bayard*
Tm of carcass samples *Nina Gardiner / Dom Bayard/ Theresa Brennan*
Improving Meat Quality in Brazilian Native Cattle *Aaron Cooper/ Ben Guimarães*
Tm effects of feeding fermented TMR to Thai Cattle *S Lloyd/ K Sommart*

Conference Dinner, Paparazzi Mandurah

Guest Speakers:
Craig McLure - Experience at CYO Incubators and Beyond
Jeremy Dawkins - Building Research Communities
Aaron Cooper - US v Australian Wagyu
John Hartley - Food and Water Security

Friday 14th July

Symposium 4: DNA testing; farm or laboratory?

Empowering Agricultural Manufacturers through fit for purpose testing methodologies *Doug Hall*
Breed Certification *Roger Dawkins*
Qiagen technologies for Johnes testing *David Reynolds*
Cutting Edge Genomics – setting up a farm Laboratory *Dom Bayard*
Applications of histology image analysis to assessing marbling in beef *Louise Smyth*

Symposium 5: Improving Pasture

Improving on Rhodes grass (managing pasture on a pastoral lease) *Chad Mitchelmore*
Value of irrigated forages for rangeland beef production systems *Clint Revell*
Genetic and Phenotypic variation of Western Australian Kikuyu varieties *Tony Lloyd*
Transposable elements in Barley *Chengdao Li*
Improved Legume Pastures *John Howieson*
Milk production on Irrigated Sorghum *Rob Giura*

Symposium 6: Sun, wind and water, powering regional development

Integrating Solar in Agriculture in WA *Ray Wills*
Solar Irrigation Systems *Rob Guira*
Energy Storage – Salt Water Battery *Manickam Minakshi*
Water management in the Peel Region *Richard Harper*

Symposium 7: Collaborations and Grant Applications

Protection of National Intellectual Property rights *Amanda McAlpine*
Future MLA Projects *Roger Dawkins*
Cattle management from the Cloud *Chris Hinks*

Saturday 15th July: Practical Systems Training in Stockbook

Session 1: Introduction and principles of Stockbook database.

Creating, Finding and identifying Animals.
Implementing and Processing treatments
Preparing for a yard session
Using the mobile app
Bulk changes and movements

Session 2: Practical Systems in the Yards

Cattle ID and weighing in the crush
Recording activities and treatments
Recording observations and measurements
Replacing missing RFID tags
Critical information and alerts
Drafting systems

2:00-4:00 Session 3: Melaleuka Farm Laboratory

Accessing and importing from other databases *Sally Lloyd*
Business and data analyses with Stockbook *Theresa Brennan*

Participants:

Prof Roger L Dawkins – Chairman, CYO Foundation (and Melaleuka Stud)
Mr Dom Bayard – Global Reproductive Solutions/ Cutting Edge Genomics
Mr Anthony Lloyd, Vice Chairman, CYO Foundation
Dr Sally S Lloyd, Director Research Laboratories
Dr Sam Dawkins, CYO Foundation Member
Dr Herbert Rebhan, DAFA, CYO Board
Mr John R Dawkins – Tillbrook Melaleuka Group
Mr Lindsay Baker – Manager, Melaleuka Stud
Dr Jose Valenzuela, CYO and Melaleuka Stud
Mr Ben Dawkins - CYO Foundation Board
Mr. Rob Giura- Peel Dairy Farming, Nth Dandalup- CYO Foundation Board
Dr Louise Smyth – University of Notre Dame/ Murdoch University
Prof Dave Pethick - Murdoch University
Prof Richard Harper – Murdoch University
Dr Lisolette Pannier – Murdoch University
Amanda McAlpine Meat and Livestock Australia
Mark Morton – Practical Systems
Teresa Brennan - Jamorrie Wagyu
Josh Sweeney – Milne Feed

Roban-Lynne Clarke – AusIndustry
Dr Russell Lyons – University of Queensland Animal Genetics Laboratory
Doug Hall – Pastoralists and Graziers Association WA
David Reynolds – Application Specialist, Qiagen
Brett Blanchett – Pardoo Station
Dr Aaron Cooper – 33 Ventures, San Angelo, TX
Mr. Adrian Pitsikas -Greenacres Turf, Serpentine
Mr. Graemme Brickwood, Serpentine Transport
Mr Alan Peggs – Pastoral Consultant,WA/ Pardoo Station
Mr Renny Lee Steere - CYO Foundation Board
Mr Wayne Cox - CYO Foundation Board
Mr Patrick Dawkins - CYO Foundation Board
Mr. Bruce Campbell – Peel Livestock Farming
Ms Paula Pownall – Grubs Up
Dr Hillary Nath – EcoAdvise

12th-14th October: Meat Quality

Welcome to the Centre for Innovation in Agriculture*Roger Dawkins*
Muscle Development *Roger Dawkins*
Centre for Innovative Agriculture: Capacity and Services *Tony Lloyd*
Centre for Innovative Agriculture: Goals and Opportunities *David Morrison*

Symposium 1: Biology of Muscle and Intra-muscular fat

Lipid metabolism and Fat Deposition *Sally Lloyd*
Biology of Marbling *Dom Bayard*

Symposium 2: Measurements to improve meat quality

World's Smallest Engine *Sam Dawkins*
Tm and Marbling *Sally Lloyd*
In Vivo Analysis of IMF Disposition *Jose L.Valenzuela*

Symposium 3: Ruminant Feeding

Ruminant Biology *Sally Lloyd*
Feeding for Fertility *Barbara Spandern*
Melaleuka Feed Trials *John Dawkins/Lindsay Baker*

Symposium 4: International Perspectives

Marbling in cattle breeds *Aaron Cooper*
Gyulais Cattle *Daniel Hammond*
Wagyu in Japan *John Dawkins*

Conference Dinner, CY O'Connor Tavern, Piara Waters

Guest Speakers:

David Morrison: Welcome

Aaron Cooper: International Cooperation for genetic improvement

Barbara Spandern: Future-proofing farms in Europe

Sam Dawkins: International Mittelstand for Incubation

Friday 14th October

Symposium 5: Improving Pasture

Pastures for the Peel Region *Rob Giura*

Productive crops for the Pilbra *Lawrence Kirton*

Grazing in the Wheatbelt *Tony Lloyd*

Optimising the soil microbiome to enhance productivity *Sofie De Meyer*

Barley for Beef and Beer. *Chengdao Li*

Symposium 6: Student presentations and Innovation Awards

Crickets for Ruminant feed *Paula Pownall*

Consumer responses to low Tm Beef *Emily Tomsett*

Marbled Wagyu on grass *Theresa Brennan*

Measuring pasture quality *Joanne Rollinson*

Effects of stress on health and productivity of cattle *Joshua Aleri*

To be announced *Herb Rovey*

Aesthetic Parameters of a Smile *Cindy Mograve*

Tour of Farm and Laboratory facilities

Retreat participants were given a tour of the farm and laboratory facilities and future sites.

Saturday 15th October

Artificial Insemination and Embryo Transfer Demonstrations

Embryo Flushing,

Embryo assessment, Embryo splitting, Embryo biopsy,

Fresh Embryo transfer

Demonstrators: *Dom Bayard, Barbara Spandern, Aaron Cooper*

Students: *Joanne Rollinson, Jose Valenzuela, Theresa Brennan*

Workshop Stockbook and Haplotype Reporting

Agenda

1) Shared CYO Lab – CEG Stockbook database
2) Haplotype and DNA test records in Stockbook
3) Intro to creating and using customised reports in Stockbook
4) CEG/CYO procedures for cross checking and entering DNA results and correcting pedigrees
5) Content of CEG Haplotyping, Paternity and Tm/Marbling reports
6) Whole genome amplification

Participants: *Sally Lloyd, Dom Bayard, Darren Hamblin, Jose Valenzuela, Aaron Cooper*

Speakers

Mr Lindsay Baker – Manager, Melaleuka Stud
Mr Dom Bayard – GRS / Cutting Edge Genomics
Mr Brett Blanchett – Pardoo Station
Ms Teresa Brennan - Jamorrie Wagyu
Mr Bruce Cheung – Pardoo Station
Dr Aaron Cooper – 33 Ventures, San Angelo, TX
Mr Ben Dawkins - CYO Foundation Board
Dr Sam Dawkins, CYO Foundation Member
Prof Roger L Dawkins – Chairman, CYO Foundation (and Melaleuka Stud)
Mr John R Dawkins – Tillbrook Melaleuka Group
Prof Graham Gardner – Murdoch Univeristy
Mr Neil Garnett
Mr Rob Giura – Peel Dairy Farming, Nth Dandalup- CYO Foundation Board
Mr Doug Hall – Pastoralists and Graziers Association WA
Prof Richard Harper – Murdoch University
Major General John Hartley (Retd) – Future Directions
Prof Chengdao Li – Murdoch University
Mr Anthony Lloyd, Vice Chairman, CYO Foundation
Dr Sally S Lloyd, Director CYO Research Laboratories
Roban-Lynne Clarke – AusIndustry
Dr Russell Lyons – University of Queensland Animal Genetics Laboratory
Amanda McAlpine – Meat and Livestock Australia
Dean Maugham – Milne Feeds
Dr Sofie De Meyer – Murdoch University
Prof David Morrison - Deputy Vice Chancellor Research and Innovation -Murdoch University

Mark Morton – Practical Systems
Dr Lisolette Pannier – Murdoch University
Prof Dave Pethick - Murdoch University
Dr Herbert Rebhan, DAFA, CYO Board
David Reynolds – Application Specialist, Qiagen
Dr Luke Robinson - CEO Sunfish Energy Limited
Ms Joanne Rollinson – CY O'Connor Foundation
Dr Louise Smyth – University of Notre Dame/ Murdoch University
Dr Barbara Spandern
Dr Josh Sweeney – Milne Feed
Ms Emily Tomsett
Dr Jose Valenzuela, CYO and Melaleuka Stud

Additional participants

Russell Lyon
Craig McLure
Malcom Mackay
Geoff Manning
Manickam Minakshi
Chad Mitchelmore
Dr Hillary Nath – Eco Advise
Matthew Nippierd
Veronica Nix
Rod Peak
Mr Alan Peggs - Pastoral Consultant,WA/ Pardoo Station
Mr. Adrian Pitsikas- Greenacres Turf, Serpentine
Ms Paula Pownall - Grubs Up
Michael Roberts
Mark Ross
Louise A Smyth
Darryl Spargo
Mr Renny Lee Steere -CYO Foundation Board
David Stoate
Josh Sweeney
Lisolette Pannier
Jason Wallis
Brian Walker
Joseph Williamson
Lindsay Wolrige
Mr. Graemme Brickwood, Serpentine Transport
Peter Bates
Theresa Brennan
Simon Brockman
Linda and David Brumby
Mick Cabassi
Mr. Bruce Campbell – Peel Livestock Farming
Roban-Lynne Clarke
Tim Connoley
Mr Wayne Cox - CYO Foundation Board
Lance Cumming
Mr Patrick Dawkins - CYO Foundation Board
Sam Dwyer
Graham Elliott
Kathy Elliott
Fiona Fiest
Nina Gardner
Ken Gordan
Valerie Gordan
Doug Hall
Richard Harper
Darren Hamblin
Steve Hills

Retreats

John Howieson
Daniel Hammond
Rick Hunter
Brett Flugge Shire of Murray
Hammond Keith
Chanvit Leelayuwat
Susan Lester
Aaron Locicero
Kate Loud

Visitors

Dr Aaron Cooper teaching farm staff how to assess young bulls

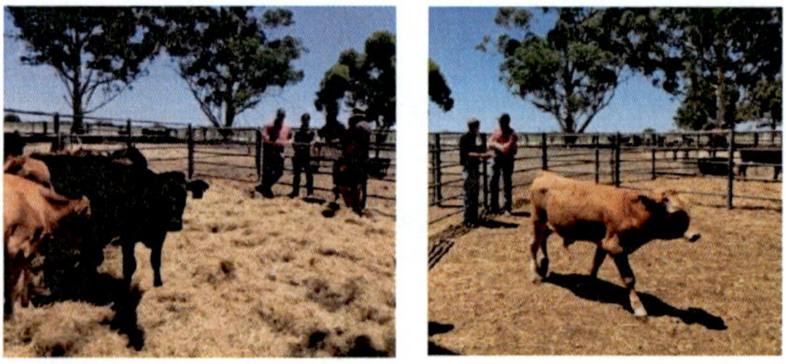

Made in United States
North Haven, CT
07 November 2026

21928341R00084